CLAIRE B. KEANE, R.N., B.S.
AND
SYBIL M. FLETCHER, R.N.

SECOND EDITION

DRUGS
AND
SOLUTIONS

A Programed Introduction for Nurses

W. B. SAUNDERS COMPANY
PHILADELPHIA • LONDON • TORONTO

W. B. Saunders Company: West Washington Square
Philadelphia, Pa.   19105

12 Dyott Street
London, WC1A   1DB

1835 Yonge Street
Toronto 7, Canada

Drugs and Solutions   SBN 0-7216-5341-3

Print No: 9   8   7   6   5   4

INTRODUCTION

The material in this textbook is programed. If you have never used a programed text before, you will be in for a few surprises when you settle down to the business of using this one to learn about the dosages of drugs and solutions.

First of all, you will have to use this text—not just read it. You must actively participate in the programed exercises we have set up for you. In fact, that is the chief purpose of any programed text: the active participation of the learner.

Second, we hope that you will accept this material in the spirit in which it was written; that is, that learning can be both exciting and rewarding when we are truly interested in achieving the goals we have set for ourselves, and when we are willing to put forth the effort necessary to reach these goals.

The content of this programed text is broken down into short, logically organized units called *frames*. Each frame asks you a question; and this is where your participation comes in. You must try to answer each question as best you can before moving on to the next one. If you have read the frame carefully (and if we have written it clearly!), you should have no trouble answering the question. The correct answer for each frame appears in a special column beside the question frame. Each frame is numbered, and the same number indentifies its answer. Tear off the perforated "slider" attached to the back cover of the book and use it to mask the printed answers until you have written out your own. You can write your answers either in the blank spaces in the program itself or on a separate sheet of paper—but whichever method you use, it is most important that you actually *write* your answers down, and not just "think" them.

Since we have given you the correct answers to every question, we obviously are not trying to trick you or test you. You will receive the greatest benefit from this program by being entirely honest with yourself, and by freely recognizing when you don't understand something and have written a wrong answer. You can then go on to the special frames we have written for those who don't get the correct answer on the first try.

For a little practice, try these two frames:

A

question

A

Programed instruction gives the student information in short, easy-to-read steps. The learner reads the information, and then answers a question about it. In each frame, the reader is asked to make an active response by answering a _____.

B

speed

B

Each person is an individual who learns in a unique way and at her own rate of speed. Some learn more rapidly than others, and some can recall things they have learned in the past more efficiently than others. The material in this text is presented so that some students can skip over material they already know.

Each student using this program can progress at her own individual rate of _____.

That was easy, wasn't it? In fact, you may have found it too *simple*—but don't let yourself become complacent. We expect you to *think* as you read each frame of the text. Then, at the end of each Part, we will give you a review test so that you can be sure that you thoroughly understand the information you have been given. This material is essential to your becoming a skilled nurse. Accept each question with that in mind—and as a challenge to you as an intelligent, thinking person: the only kind of person who can make a real contribution to nursing.

A NOTE TO THE INSTRUCTOR

One of the greatest challenges in writing programed instruction is that it requires the writer to establish a clear, precise picture of what he expects the student to learn. Before we undertook this program, we set up for ourselves the objectives that follow. We would encourage you as an instructor to read the objectives we have outlined because they present in specific terms the goals and purposes of this text.

This text should not be used as one would use a conventional text. Programed instruction is designed primarily for *self-instruction*. Each student should be allowed to work independently at her own pace. The function of the instructor is to provide help in areas in which the student may have difficulty or to supplement the material with information pertinent to what the student is learning.

In this second edition we have revised the post-tests to include more nursing situations and have added a complete final examination set on perforated pages so that it can be removed and later distributed to the students as an actual test. It was requested by many of our readers that we add tables; these can be found inside the front and back covers. We have also included some illustrations to help the reader who is not familiar with the equipment used in administering drugs and solutions.

The suggestions and criticisms we have received from our readers have helped to make the second edition more concise and, we hope, more effective for the student and the instructor.

A STATEMENT OF OBJECTIVES

1.   The learner should be able to name and describe the three systems of measurement used in the weighing and measuring of drugs and solutions.

2.   Given a list of the various symbols and abbreviations used to express units of weight and measure in the three systems, the learner should be able to read and interpret these symbols and abbreviations correctly.

3.   Provided with a list of specific quantities of medications, the learner should be able to write each of the dosages using the proper symbols, abbreviations, and numbers.

4.   Given a list of the more commonly used units of weight and measure in the apothecaries', metric, and household systems, the learner should be able to identify the system from which each unit is taken and give its approximate equivalent in the other systems of measurement.

5.   Presented with situations in which dosage is ordered in one system of measurement, and is available only in another system, the learner should be able to demonstrate a ready knowledge of conversion by calculating the correct amount of drug to be given the patient.

6.   Given a group of situations in which a small amount of solution for parenteral administration must be prepared from a powdered drug, the learner should be aware of the necessity for reading the instructions provided by the manufacturer and for following these instructions precisely when adding the proper

amount of diluent to obtain the correct dosage.

7. Confronted with a group of situations in which a small amount of solution must be prepared from hypodermic tablets, the learner should be able to determine the number of tablets to be dissolved and the amount of diluent necessary to obtain the correct dosage.

8. Given a group of situations in which dosage must be calculated from a stock solution, the learner should be able to set up each problem according to ratio and proportion, and determine the correct amount of solution to be given.

9. Provided with a group of situations in which the drug ordered is dispensed in units, the learner should be able to calculate the correct dosage to be given from the amount on hand.

10. Given a group of situations in which the dosage of insulin must be administered from a 2-cc or tuberculin syringe, the learner should be able to determine the number of milliliters or minims the patient is to receive.

11. Given a group of situations in which a large amount of solution must be prepared from a pure drug, the learner should be able to set up a proportion for the purpose of determining the amount of pure drug to be dissolved in a given amount of diluent to achieve the correct concentration in each instance.

12. Provided with a group of theoretical situations in which a large amount of solution must be prepared from a stock solution, the learner should be able to set up a proportion for each situation, and to determine the amount of stock solution to be added to a given amount of diluent to achieve the correct strength in each instance.

CONTENTS

PART ONE   INTRODUCTION TO SYSTEMS OF
               MEASUREMENT.. 1

     Post-Test 5

PART TWO   THE APOTHECARIES' SYSTEM.................... 7

     UNIT I
     UNITS OF MEASURE IN THE APOTHECARIES'
     SYSTEM 8

     UNIT II
     ABBREVIATIONS, SYMBOLS, AND NUMBERS IN THE
     APOTHECARIES' SYSTEM 17

     UNIT III
     REVIEW OF FRACTIONS 25

     Post-Test 54

PART THREE   THE HOUSEHOLD SYSTEM 57

PART FOUR   THE METRIC SYSTEM................................. 61

     UNIT I
     REVIEW OF DECIMALS 62

UNIT II
UNITS OF MEASURE IN THE METRIC SYSTEM 79

UNIT III
*ABBREVIATIONS, SYMBOLS, AND NUMBERS IN THE
METRIC SYSTEM* 82

UNIT IV
*EXCHANGING WEIGHTS WITHIN THE METRIC
SYSTEM* 85

Post-Test 91

PART FIVE   EXCHANGING UNITS OF WEIGHT AND
MEASURE BETWEEN THE
APOTHECARIES' AND THE METRIC
SYSTEMS 95

UNIT I
EXCHANGING UNITS OF MEASURE 96

UNIT II
EXCHANGING UNITS OF WEIGHT 103

Post-Test 115

PART SIX   PREPARING SOLUTIONS FOR
PARENTERAL ADMINISTRATION 117

UNIT I
POWDERED DRUGS 118

UNIT II
HYPODERMIC TABLETS 121

UNIT III
STOCK SOLUTIONS 125

UNIT IV
DRUGS MEASURED IN UNITS 129

UNIT V
CALCULATING INSULIN DOSAGE 133

Post-Test 139

PART SEVEN   PREPARING LARGE AMOUNTS OF
SOLUTIONS 141

    UNIT I
    PURE DRUGS 142

    UNIT II
    STOCK SOLUTIONS 152

    Post-Test 159

ANSWERS TO THE POST-TEST QUESTIONS 160

EXAMINATION 167

ANSWERS TO THE EXAMINATION QUESTIONS 171

PART ONE

INTRODUCTION TO SYSTEMS OF MEASUREMENT

1

In the early history of drug preparation, medicines were administered in the form of powders or brews made from herbs, roots and other parts of plants. There was no way of knowing exactly *how much* medication a patient was receiving, because no standards had been set for accurately weighing and measuring drugs.

Today, when a physician prescribes a drug, he is assured of the accuracy of the dosage because there are universally accepted standards or systems for the measurement of drugs.

2

system
measurement

A universally accepted standard which assures accuracy in the weighing and measuring of drugs is called a _____. of _____.

3

apothecaries'

In the United States we now use two systems of measurement in preparing and administering drugs. Of the two, the *apothecaries'* system is the older. It was brought to the United States from England during the colonial period.

A system of measurement brought to the United States in the eighteenth century, and still used today in the preparation and administration of drugs, is the

_____ system.

4

metric

4

Another system by which drugs are weighed and measured is the metric system. This system is more convenient than the apothecaries' system, and it is the one used in the official listings of drugs.

Since most drugs are prepared and dispensed from an official listing, the system most frequently used in the weighing and measuring of drugs is the

_____ system.

5

apothecaries'
metric (either
order)

5

Two systems used for weighing and measuring drugs in the United States are the _____ system and the _____ system.

6

6

The administration of drugs would be much simpler if all drugs were prescribed, weighed, measured, and dispensed according to one universal system of measurement. However, even though the apothecaries' system is gradually being replaced by the metric system, each system is in current use, and the nurse must be familiar with both.

apothecaries'
metric

Sometimes a physician will prescribe a dosage of a drug using the apothecaries' system, when the drug is dispensed according to the units of the metric system. When this happens, the nurse must be able to translate, or convert, from units of measure in the _____ system to units of measure in the _____ system.

7

household

7

Drugs such as milk of magnesia, cough syrup and other medications sold in drug stores and administered in the home as well as in the hospital are usually measured and administered in a household article such as a teaspoon or a tablespoon. Although these articles do not give so completely accurate a measurement as the metric and apothecaries' systems, they are recognized and used as units of measure in the household system.

Another system of measurement used for measuring drugs commonly sold in drug stores and taken in the home is the _____ system.

POST-TEST ON SYSTEMS OF MEASUREMENT

Write the correct word or words to complete each of the following statements:

1. A universally accepted standard which assures accuracy in weighing and measuring drugs is called a
_____ of measurement.

2. The two principal systems used for weighing and measuring drugs in the United States are the
_____ system and the _____
system.

3. A system of measurement which is not completely accurate but is sometimes used for administering medications in the home is the _____
system.

4. The system of measurement used most often in preparing and dispensing drugs is the_____
system.

5. An older system of measurement that is frequently used by physicians in prescribing drugs is the _____
system.

PART TWO

THE APOTHECARIES' SYSTEM

UNIT I

UNITS OF MEASURE IN THE APOTHECARIES' SYSTEM

1

units
measure

1

Before we can understand any system of measurement, we must have some concept of the *units* of measure in that system. For example, inches, feet, and yards are units of linear measure.

When the nurse administers drugs prescribed in the apothecaries' system, she must be familiar with the _____ of _____ in that system.

2

apothecaries'

2

Americans are familiar with many of the units of measure in the apothecaries' system because we use them in our everyday life. We buy gasoline by the gallon, milk by the quart, and cream by the pint. The gallon, the quart, and the pint are all units of measure in the_____ system.

3

12 irrigations

3

Now try this problem: A nurse in central supply prepared 3 gallons of Zephiran solution for vaginal irrigations. If each irrigation requires 1 quart of Zephiran solution, then 3 gallons of the solution would be sufficient for_____irrigations.

If your answer was correct, please go on to Frame 6. If you did not get the correct answer or are not sure how the answer was obtained go to Frame 4.

4

12 irrigations

4

Perhaps you don't know the apothecaries' system as well as we thought. There are 4 quarts in 1 gallon. Three gallons of solution would be sufficient for 3×4 or _____ irrigations.

5

2 one-gallon jugs

5

Now see if you can get this one. If we needed to prepare 8 quarts of a sterile solution in one-gallon containers, it would be necessary to sterilize · 2 one-gallon jugs / 4 one-gallon jugs · before preparing the solution.

6

2 quarts

6

Let us suppose that a nurse must prepare enough saline solution for 4 irrigations during the day. If she will need 1 pint of saline solution for each irrigation, she should prepare · 1 quart / 2 quarts · of the solution. If your answer came out 1 quart, please go on to Frame 7; if it was 2 quarts, go on to Frame 8.

7

2 quarts

7

You must have forgotten that 2 pints are equal to 1 quart. If there are 2 pints in 1 quart, then 4 pints would be equal to _____ quart(s).

8

quart
pint
ounce (or fluid ounce)

8

The next smaller unit in the apothecaries' system, after the pint, is the *fluid* ounce. Most people are familiar with the word ounce used in relation to the weighing of solids; however, the nurse will most often see ounce used in measuring liquid drugs. The measurement may be written as ounce or *fluid* ounce. Either term is correct.

In descending order of size, the units of the apothecaries' system for measuring liquids are: the gallon, the_____ the _____ , and the _____.

9

quart

gallon

1 quart

9

You now know four units of measure in the apothecaries' system: the ounce, the pint, the_____ , and the_____.

There are 32 ounces in 1 quart. If an infant is receiving 4 ounces of formula per feeding, you would need to prepare_____ quart(s) of formula for 8 feedings.

10

4 1/2 quarts

10

If a child drinks 6 eight-ounce glasses of milk each day, you will need_____ quart(s) for a three-day supply.

If you answered this correctly, go on to Frame 13. If you don't see how we got this figure, go on to Frame 11.

11

4 1/2 quarts

11

There are two steps in this problem. First, you must determine the total number of ounces the child will drink in *one* day (6x8 ounces = (equal) 48 ounces). A three-day supply would be 3x48 ounces, or 144 ounces. To change ounces to quarts, you would divide this number by 32 (because there are 32 ounces in a quart). Therefore your answer is _____ quart(s).

12

2 1/4 quarts

12

A physician orders milk and cream for a patient with a peptic ulcer. The dosage is 3 ounces every hour. If you were responsible for ordering the milk and cream from the diet kitchen every morning, you would order_____ quart(s) of the mixture for a 24-hour period.

13

1 1/2 quarts

13

Suppose that you are caring for a patient who receives 4 ounces of tube feeding every 2 hours. Since the tube feeding is prepared in quarts and is ordered only once a day from the diet kitchen, you would order_____ quart(s) for a 24-hour period.

14

14

1 pint

Weak and debilitated patients sometimes receive dietary supplements to increase their intake of food elements. Sustagen is the name of one such dietary supplement, and a prescription for it is usually filled in the diet kitchen. If a physician orders 4 ounces to be given 4 times a day, the dietitian would expect the nurse to order_____pint(s) for a one-day supply.

15

15

dram

When we measure liquids we usually choose the unit of measure that most nearly represents the amount we need. Thus, if we need large amounts, we measure the liquid in quarts rather than ounces: and if we need smaller amounts, we use ounces rather than quarts. Should we need to measure an even smaller amount, we could use drams.

In the apothecaries' system, a unit of measure that is smaller than the ounce is the_____.

16

16

The standard medicine glass used in many hospitals for the administration of liquid medication by mouth is a one-ounce glass. This small glass is usually marked, or graduated, in drams. Sometimes the glass is graduated in ounces, drams, and other units.

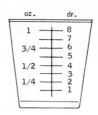

8 drams

In the drawing, you can see that 1 ounce is equal to_____dram(s).

17

4 drams

17

If a physician orders 1/2 ounce of medication for a patient, you would give the patient_____dram(s).

18

16 drams

18

Sometimes a physician will order 2 ounces of a certain medication. This is equal to approximately_____dram(s).

19

minim

19

Another unit of measure in the apothecaries' system is the *minim*. The word *minim* means "the least."

The smallest unit of liquid measure in the apothecaries' system is the_____.

20

minims
minim

20

When a minim is used as a unit of measure, it is usually because the drug to be administered is very potent. When such a drug is to be given by injection, prepare it in a syringe graduated in _____.
If the drug is ordered for oral administration, however, it should be measured in a_____ glass.

21

should never

21

To form some idea of the amount represented by a minim, you might compare the minim to a drop. Drops vary greatly in size, however, and this is a most inaccurate comparison. If the physician prescribes a drug in minims, the nurse · can usually/ should never · substitute I drop for 1 minim.

22

60 minims

22

The drawing below shows a minim glass used to administer minute portions of a medication by mouth. The glass is graduated in both minims and drams.

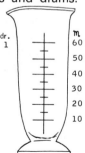

You can see that I dram is equal to approximately_____minims.

23

30 minims

23

If a physician orders 1/2 dram of a certain medication, it could be measured in a minim glass. One-half dram is equal to approximately_____minims.

24

20 minims

24

Minim glasses are not always available to the nurse and so she may need to use a syringe for an accurate measurement of an oral drug prescribed in fractions of a dram. Look at the 2-cc. syringe below.

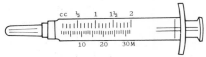

If a physician ordered 1/3 of a dram of medication, the nurse would give the patient_____minims.

25

1/2 dram

25

A patient with emphysema is to receive 10 minims of saturated solution of potassium iodide three times a day. A total amount of _____dram(s) is given each day.

26

26

Most textbooks on drugs and solutions contain a number of tables of equivalents. It is not necessary for you to memorize all of these tables, because you already know some equivalents of liquid measure in the apothecaries' system from working the previous problems.

How many equivalents do you already know in the following table?

Fluid measure in the apothecaries' system

4 quarts	_____ quarts	= 1 gallon
2 pints	_____ pints	= 1 quart
32 ounces	_____ ounces	= 1 quart
8 drams	_____ drams	= 1 ounce
60 minims	_____ minims	= 1 dram

27

solid

27

All the units in the Table in Frame 26. pertained to liquid measure. There is, however, one unit of weight in the apothecaries' system that is still used quite frequently for solid drugs, and it should be included here. This unit of weight originally was compared to a grain of wheat, and is very conveniently called a grain.

In the apothecaries' system the quart, the ounce, and the dram are three units used in measuring liquids; the grain is a unit sometimes used in weighing _____ drugs.

28

grain

28

Although there are many other units of weight in the apothecaries' system, the grain is the only one that a nurse is likely to use.

Since all the other units have become generally obsolete, the only unit of weight in the apothecaries' system that we will be concerned with here is the _____ .

UNIT II

ABBREVIATIONS, SYMBOLS, AND NUMBERS IN THE APOTHECARIES' SYSTEM

1

1

You have probably been in nursing school long enough to realize that physicians and nurses speak and write a language all their own. You have struggled through Latin prefixes and suffixes, trying to make some sense out of medical terminology—but brace yourself, there is more to come! There are also a number of abbreviations and symbols that you must know before you can give medications to your patients.

2

gallon . . . . . . gal.
quart . . . . . . qt.
pint . . . . . . pt.
ounce . . . . . . oz.

2

Don't get discouraged! Things really aren't as bad as we have suggested. You are already familiar with some of the abbreviations used for units of measure in the apothecaries' system. Look at the list below and see how well you can do:

Unit of measure	Abbreviation
gallon	_____
quart	_____
pint	_____
ounce	_____

If you missed any of the abbreviations in Frame 2, go back and study them carefully. We will use these abbreviations often in the frames to come.

3

3

gr.

The abbreviations for dram and grain are easy. We just use the first two letters of the word and then put a period at the end. Therefore, the abbreviation for dram is dr., and the abbreviation for grain is_____.

4

4

the symbol

In the preceding frames we learned a few abbreviations, but we did not say anything about symbols. Symbols are letters or signs that are used as substitutes for an entire word. The sign ℥ is · the symbol / an abbreviation · for ounce.

5

5

℥

The symbol for ounce is ℥. The symbol for dram is ʒ. Because they are so similar, it is important to avoid confusing the two. In charting medications on a patient's medical record, the nurse should use the symbol · ʒ / ℥ · to designate ounce.

6

6

ʒ

If a physician orders a medication in drams, you would use the symbol_____in charting the medication.

7

minim

7

The symbol for minim is easy to remember because it resembles a small m. It is written like this: ℳ If you saw a small glass marked with the symbol ℳ, you would know that it was a _____ glass.

8

Roman numerals

8

You remember that we have called the apothecaries' system a very old system of measurement. You also know that Roman numerals have been used for counting since ancient times. It would be fairly safe, then, to guess that the numbers used to designate amounts in the apothecaries' system would be _____ .

9

9

Reading Roman numerals should be nothing new to you. They are used in chapter headings, on clocks and sundials, and in many other places. Since you will be using small Roman numerals in reading prescriptions and charting dosages of drugs, test yourself on the following:

	Roman numeral	Arabic number
1	i	_____
4	iv	_____
5	v	_____
7	vii	_____
9	ix	_____
10	x	_____
22	xxii	_____
34	xxxiv	_____

If you missed any of the small Roman numerals in Frame 9, you should go on to Frame 10 and review them. If all your answers were right, go on to Frame 18.

10

xv

10

We are going to consider only the Roman numerals that designate the smaller a- mounts, because these are the only ones that a nurse will use in reading physician's orders and charting medications. The two most important numerals to remember are x and v. The x represents 10 and the v represents 5. If we combine x and v, We get 15. The Roman numeral for 15 is._____

11

added to

11

We can see that by writing v to the right of x we have added v, which is 5, to x, which is 10. When a numeral follows one of larger value, it is · added to / subtracted from · the numeral it follows.

12

12

three

The smaller Roman numerals other than x and v are easy to read. The i is one, ii is two, and iii is_____.

13

13

13

If the smaller numerals to the right are always added to the numeral of larger value, then xiii is the same as the Arabic number _____.

14

14

9

We have seen that the position of one Roman numeral in relation to another is very important. Whenever a smaller numeral follows one of larger value, the numerals are added. But if a smaller numeral precedes one of larger value, it is subtracted from the larger numeral. Therefore, ix means 10 minus 1, or_____.

15

15

4

You know that i is less than v. The Roman numeral iv, therefore, represents the Arabic number_____.

16

16

30

Sometimes we see a combination of Roman numerals that are of equal value; for example, xxx. When the numerals are written this way, all their values are added. Thus, xxx equals $10+10+10$, or_____.

8
16
24
35
14

17

Let's go through another set of Roman numerals and their Arabic equivalents, to be sure you understand them thoroughly:

Roman numeral	Arabic number
viii	_____
xvi	_____
xxiv	_____
xxxv	_____
xiv	_____

ss.

18

To express parts of a unit in the apothecaries' system, we use common fractions such as 2/3 or 3/4. The only exception to this rule is 1/2, which is expressed by the Latin abbreviation ss.

When we wish to express the fraction 1/2 in the apothecaries' system, we use the abbreviation_____.

℥ ii

19

There is one more thing you should know about writing weights and measures in the apothecaries' system. That is, that the numbers indicating the amount to be given are always written *after* the symbol or abbreviation for the unit of measure. If you were charting 2 ounces of a medication, you would write it as_____. (Be sure to use the symbol for ounce.)

20

2 1/2 ounces

20

Now you should be ready to read and write any unit of measure in the apothecaries' system according to the rules you have learned.

Let's say that a physician orders milk of magnesia ℥ iiss. This should be read as

_____.

21

1 1/2 ounces

21

If a physician orders mineral oil ℥ iss., you would give the patient _____ of the drug.

22

4 ounces

22

If the medicine card reads ℥ iv, you would pour _____ of the medication.

23

℥ iii

23

Suppose you were instructed to give 3 ounces of a certain medication. In charting this you would write the symbol and amount as _____.

24

2 drams

24

An order reading cascara ʒ ii means that the patient is to receive _____ of cascara.

25

ʒ i

25

If a physician orders 1 dram of Elixir of Donnatal, you would chart the symbol and amount as _____.

26

12 minims

26

Suppose that you have an order written: tincture of belladonna ♏ xii. You should read the amount as_____.

27

♏ iv

27

If a physician orders 4 minims of a certain drug, you would chart this amount as _____.

28

gr. 1/4

28

Here we run into some difficulty with the apothecaries' system, and can sympathize with those who wish to do away with it. We have said that Roman numerals are used in the apothecaries' system and that parts of a whole are expressed as common fractions. The Romans, however, had no way of expressing fractions such as 1/4 and 1/8 in numbers. In fact, the only common fraction we can indicate in Latin is 1/2, which is abbreviated ss. All other common fractions must be written in Arabic numbers.

Therefore, to express 1/4 grain, you would write gr._____.

UNIT III
REVIEW OF FRACTIONS

1

1

Inconvenient as the apothecaries' system may be, we are still using it, and the nurse must know fractions and how to use them in calculations if she is going to administer medications intelligently.

The word fraction indicates one or more equal parts of a unit. If a unit is divided into two or more equal parts, the parts of the unit are referred to, and written, as fractions.

2

2

$4 \div 6$

In the fraction 4/6, the line between the two numbers is read "divided by." You could write 4/6 as_____ ÷ _____.

3

3

3
3

The number below the fraction line indicates the way a unit is divided, and is called the denominator. Look at this drawing:

Since the unit (the whole circle) has been divided into_____parts, the denominator of the fraction is_____.

4

smaller

5

smaller

6

less

7

1
3

4

We know that the denominator indicates the way a unit is divided, and also that the more we divide a unit the smaller the parts will be. In other words, the larger the denominator, the · smaller / larger · the size of each part.

5

The fraction 1/300 represents a · larger / smaller · amount than 1/100.

6

Suppose that you needed to give a patient gr. 1/8 of morphine sulfate, and the only tablets on hand were gr. 1/4 tablets. Is gr. 1/8 more or less than gr. 1/4 ? _____.

7

The number above the fraction line is called the numerator, and indicates the number of parts *taken* from the unit. In the drawing, the shaded area indicates the part taken:

Here, the numerator is_____and the denominator is_____.

8

(a) proper
(b) improper
(c) mixed number

Life would be much simpler for everyone if there were only one kind of fraction. Actually there are three, and examples of each kind are given below. See if you can remember from your earlier experience with arithmetic what these are called, and write down the name of each kind of fraction beside the example given.:

(a) 1/3 _____ fraction
(b) 8/5 _____ fraction
(c) 2 1/4 _____ _____

If you got all three answers to Frame 8 correct, go on to Frame 18. If you aren't sure about these three kinds of fractions, continue with Frame 9.

9

parts

There are three types of fractions: proper fractions, improper fractions, and mixed numbers. When we think of the word "fraction," we think of a unit divided into equal parts. A proper fraction refers to the division of only one unit into two or more equal_____.

10

number
divided
numerator
denominator

We have seen that the numerator indicates the_____of equal parts taken from a unit, and that the denominator indicates the way in which the unit is_____.
In a proper fraction, the_____ cannot be larger than the_____.

11

proper

11

In a proper fraction, the denominator is always larger than the numerator. Fractions in which the numerator is *smaller* than the denominator are called_____ fractions.

12

larger

12

The opposite of proper is improper. Proper fractions have numerators that are smaller than their denominators. In improper fractions, the numerators are_____ than the denominators.

13

5/4

13

Improper fractions indicate the division of more than one unit. In the drawing below, you can see that two units have been divided into fourths. The five parts taken have been shaded. We can represent this division by writing the improper fraction_____.

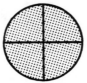 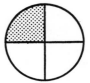

14

1/4

14

If in the drawing in Frame 13 you counted all the shaded areas together, you could say that they represented the improper fraction 5/4. If you counted these shaded areas as parts taken from *two separate* units, you could say that they represented a mixed *number*, 1 and_____.

(fraction)

15

are

15

A mixed number represents one or more whole units, plus part of another unit. An improper fraction represents parts of more than one unit. Thus, improper fractions and mixed numbers · , are / are not · . two different ways of expressing the same amount.

16

proper
mixed number
improper fraction

16

Therefore, 1/2 is a(n)_____ fraction; 1 1/2 is a(n)_____ _____; and 6/5 is a(n) _____.

17

17

There are three types of fractions: proper fractions, improper fractions, and mixed numbers. Look at the following examples and say which type each fraction represents:

(a) proper fraction   (a) 3/8 is a(n)_____

_____.

(b) mixed number   (b) 21 3/4 is a(n)_____

_____.

(c) improper   (c) 9/8 is a(n)_____
fraction
_____.

(d) mixed number   (d) 2 5/8 is a(n)_____

_____.

(e) proper fraction   (e) 13/15 is a(n)_____

_____.

18   ## 18

improper fraction   Because improper fractions and mixed
                         numbers represent two different ways of
                         expressing the same amount, it really
                         doesn't matter which we use. There are
                         times, however, when it is much easier to
                         work arithmetic problems if we write the
                         mixed number as a(n)_____

                         _____ _____.

19   ## 19

15/2   Can you change a mixed number to an
                         improper fraction? The mixed number 7 1/2
                         may be written as the improper fraction

                         _____.

                         If you feel confident in changing mixed
                         numbers to improper fractions, go on to
                         Frame 25. If you would like a review go to
                         Frame 20.

20

1×8

20

We can change any mixed number to an improper fraction by following two quick and easy steps. First we multiply the whole number by the denominator of the fraction. For instance, to change the mixed number 1 7/8 to an improper fraction, our first step would be to multiply _____ × _____.

21

15

21

We have multiplied the whole number 1 by the denominator of the fraction, 8. Now we take the result of this multiplication and add it to the our *numerator* of the fraction. After adding 8 to 7, our answer is _____ eighths.

22

40
43

22

Let's try both steps together, and change 10 3/4 to an improper fraction.

    First step: $10 \times 4 =$ _____ fourths
    Second step: add   3   fourths
    Your answer   _____ fourths

23

$12 \times 5 = 60$
add 3
answer: 63

23

Now suppose you needed to change 12 3/5 to an improper fraction.

    First: _____ × _____ = _____ fifths
    Second: add   _____ fifths
    Your answer: _____ fifths

24

(a) 21/8
(b) 11/8
(c) 20/7
(d) 41/9

24

Just for practice, change these mixed numbers to improper fractions:

(a)　2 5/8 = _____
(b)　1 3/8 = _____
(c)　2 6/7 = _____
(d)　4 5/9 = _____

25

numerator
denominator
same

25

The numerator and denominator of a fraction are called the *terms* of that fraction. Sometimes when we work with a fraction, we must change its terms. For example, we can change the terms of a fraction by multiplying or by dividing *both* terms by the same number—a process called *finding equivalent fractions.* In finding equivalent fractions, we must multiply or divide both the _____ and the _____ by the _____ number.

26

value

26

Finding an equivalent fraction does not alter the value of the fractional parts. The numbers in the numerator and denominator are changed, but the _____ of the fractional parts remains the same.

27

multiply

27

One way of making a number larger is to multiply it by another number. If we wished to find an equivalent fraction in which both terms are larger, we could _____ both terms by the same number.

28

divide
the same number

28

Multiplication makes a number larger; division makes it smaller. If we need to find an equivalent fraction in which both terms are smaller, we could _____ both terms by_____.

29

multiply
divide

29

When we want to find an equivalent fraction in which both terms are larger than those in the original fraction, we can _____ by any number. But when we want an equivalent fraction in which the terms are smaller, we must_____ by a number that will go *evenly* into both the numerator and the denominator of the original fraction.

30

equivalent
smaller

30

Finding an equivalent fraction in which both terms are smaller is sometimes called "reducing the fraction to lower terms." When we reduce a fraction to lower terms, we are finding a(n) _____ fraction that is_____.

31

multiply

Now you can see that finding an equivalent fraction can involve either reducing the fraction or enlarging it, depending on whether you divide or_____ both terms by the same number.

32

(a) 3/5
(b) 4/5
(c) cannot be further reduced
(d) 4/5
(e) cannot be further reduced

For practice in finding equivalent fractions in which both terms are smaller, reduce the following fraction to their lowest terms:

(a)	9/15	_____
(b)	12/15	_____
(c)	5/8	_____
(d)	16/20	_____
(e)	3/16	_____

33

gr. 6/6 = 1 grain

You're ready now to get down to the business of adding fractions. Try this problem to see how well you do: A patient has received the following doses of a certain drug—gr. 1/3, gr. 1/6 and gr. ss. (You'll recall that ss. means 1/2.) What is the total amount of drug the patient received?

_____.

The addition of fractions involves several steps. If you got the answer to Frame 33 right, you must already understand these steps and you should, therefore, go on to Frame 49. If you missed the question, or if you're unsure about it, continue with Frame 34 for a review of the addition of fractions.

34

numerators

34

When we add fractions we must remember that we are adding parts of a unit that has been divided. The numerators indicate the parts taken from the unit. In adding fractions, only the_____are added.

35

value

35

Another point to remember is that the way in which a unit has been divided determines the value or size of the parts taken. If you divided a tablet into 4 parts, and then divided a similar tablet into 2 parts, you would not consider all parts of both tablets to be of equal_____.

36

denominators

36

The denominator of a fraction shows the way in which a unit has been divided. If you wished to add the parts of several units, you would have to make sure first that all of the units had been divided in the same way. Another way of saying this is: The _____ of all the fractions to be added together must be the same.

37

denominator

37

There are two steps in the addition of fractions of like denominators. First, add the numerators, and secondly place the sum of all the numerators over the _____, which is the same for all the fractions being added.

38

5/4 grains, or gr. 1 1/4

38

The nurse uses these two steps in the addition of fractions when she needs to know the total amount of a drug her patient has received. For instance, Mrs. Jones received gr. 3/4 of a drug at 10:00 a.m., gr. 1/4 at 2:00 p.m., and gr. 1/4 at 5:00 p.m. How much of the drug did she receive during the day? (Write your answer both as an improper fraction and as a mixed number.)_____.

39

equivalent denominator

39

But what happens when the denominators are not all alike? Then you must change the fractions to _____ fractions, so that all the denominators are the same. The first step in doing this is called finding the "lowest common_____."

40

common

40

We know that a denominator that is "common to" all the denominators in the fractions being added must have some similarity to, or something in _____with, all these denominators.

41

denominators

41

The one thing it must have in common with these denominators is *divisibility.* In other words, it must be a number that can be evenly divided by the_____ of all fractions being added.

42

15

42

When you are working with small fractions, finding the lowest common denominator can usually be done just by inspection. Look at this column of fractions:

3/5
4/5
2/3

The lowest common denominator (the L.C.D.) of the fractions in this column is

_____.

43

denominators

43

If you chose 15 for the L.C.D. in Frame 42, you were right. This number can be divided evenly by the denominators 5 and 3 in the column of fractions. It is also the lowest possible number that is divisible by all the _____ in the column.

NOTE: When the L.C.D. cannot be determined by inspection, we must resort to mechanical means to determine the number. Because a nurse almost always works with small fractions, we have not included this problem in the program.

44

44

3
9

When you have determined the L.C.D., you must change all the fractions being added so that each one will have the L.C.D. figure as its denominator. We know that when the denominator is changed the numerator must also be changed, so that the value of the fraction will remain the same.

There is a quick and easy way to find the numerator. Let's say our fraction is 3/5 and the L.C.D. is 15:

First: $15 \div 5 =$ _____
Second: $3 \times 3 =$ _____

45

45

9/15

The number 9 is our new numerator. This is placed over the L.C.D., and 3/5 becomes

_____.
(fraction)

46

15 ÷ 3 = 5
5 × 2 = 10
10/15

46

We'll try this one more time with the fraction 2/3. Our L.C.D. is 15.

First: the L.C.D. is divided by the denominator:

_____ ÷ _____ = _____

Second: mulitiply this number by the numerator of the fraction:

_____ × _____ = _____

We have now changed 2/3 to_____.
                                    (fraction)

47

9/15
12/15
10/15

47

For our original column of fractions, the L.C.D. is 15. How would the fractions look after changing them so that all the denominators are 15 ?

3/5 = _____
4/5 = _____
2/3 = _____

48

31/15

48

Now you can add these fractions just as you would add any other fractions with like denominators. Thus, 9/15 + 12/15 + 10/15 = _____.

(a) 14/10
   (or 7/5)
(b) 41/24
(c) 6/4 (or 3/2)
(d) 19/12

49

Test yourself on the following problems to be sure that you understand the addition of fractions:

(a) 1/2
    3/5
   +3/10
   ――――

(b) 1/2
    3/8
   +5/6
   ――――

(c) 1/2
    1/4
   +3/4
   ――――

(d) 1/6
    2/3
   +3/4
   ――――

50

5 3/8 quarts

50

If you understand the addition of fractions, you should have no trouble with the addition of mixed numbers, because when we add mixed numbers we are simply adding whole numbers and fractions. See how well you can do with the following situations: A head nurse is checking her supply of sterile saline solution. In one bottle she has 1 1/2 quarts, in another bottle 2 3/4 quarts, and in a third bottle 1 1/8 quarts.

She has a total of _____ quart(s) of saline solution.

If you worked the problem in Frame 50 without difficulty, go on to Frame 58. If you were not sure how to work the problem, go on to Frame 51 for a review of adding mixed numbers.

51

right

51

A column of mixed numbers is very similar to a column of whole numbers with two digits, for there are actually two columns to be added. When we add either mixed numbers or numbers of two or more digits, we always add the column on the · left / right · first.

52

right
fractions

52

In a mixed number, the fraction is written to the right of the whole number. Since we always begin by adding the column on the _____, our first step in the addition of *mixed numbers* is to add the · whole numbers/fractions ·

53

fractions
whole numbers

53

When we add columns of mixed numbers, we add the _____ first and then the _____ _____.

54

mixed
whole numbers

Our third step is to add the sum of the fractions to the sum of the whole numbers. If the sum of the fractions is an improper fraction—as it often is—we must change it to a_____number before it is added to the sum of the_____

_____.

15/8

55

Now let's use these steps in a problem involving the addition of mixed numbers. The column of mixed numbers is:

$$1 \ 3/4$$
$$2 \ 5/8$$
$$+1 \ 1/2$$

The first step in adding these figures is to find the sum of the column of fractions, the column on the right. Before doing this, however, we must find the L.C.D. and change all the fractions to equivalent fractions, This gives us:

$$6/8$$
$$5/8$$
$$+4/8$$

Thus_____is your answer for the sum
   (fraction)
of the column of fractions.

56

56

1 7/8

We take the sum of the fractions and then change the resulting improper fraction to a mixed number.

$$15/8 = \underline{\hspace{2cm}}$$

57

57

5 7/8

Now we must find the sum of the whole numbers $(1 + 2 + 1 = 4)$, and add this to the sum of the fractions (1 7/8):

$$\begin{array}{r} 4 \\ +1 \ 7/8 \\ \hline \end{array}$$

Your answer: _____

58

58

(a) 6 6/15
(b) 10 7/8
(c) 15 11/24
(d) 8 5/8

Add the following mixed numbers. Be sure to find the L.C.D. and to change all the fractions to equivalent fractions of like denominators before you add them.

(a) 1 2/5   (b) 4 1/4
     3 2/3   1 1/2
    +1 5/15   +5 1/8
    _____   _____

(c) 8 1/3   (d) 1 4/16
     4 3/8   2 3/4
    +2 3/4   +4 5/8
    _____   _____

gr. 1/8

59

Now let us see how well you remember the subtraction of fractions. One of your patients is to receive gr. 1/8 of morphine sulfate, and the only dosage on hand is an ampule containing gr. 1/4. Since morphine is a narcotic, you are required to account for the amount you do not use for the patient.

gr. 1/4 − gr. 1/8 = _____ grain(s)

If you answered the question in Frame 59 correctly, go on to Frame 64. If you did not understand how to do it, go on to Frame 60 for a review of the subtraction of fractions.

common
subtract

60

When we add fractions, we can only add the numerators of fractions with like denominators. The same rule applies when we subtract fractions.

In the subtraction of fractions we must have a_____denominator before we can_____one numerator from the other.

2/8 (or 1/4)

61

Suppose that you wanted to subtract 2/8 from 4/8. That's easy, because your denominators are the same and the numbers in the numerator are so small that you can work the problem in your head. Your answer is_____.

62

5/16

62

Now let's subtract 2/8 from 9/16. The answer is · 7/8 / 5/16 ·

63

equivalent
numerators

63

Remember that we subtract only the numerators, and that all the fractions must have a common denominator. We must first find the L.C.D. and then change to _____ fractions before we can subtract the _____.

64

(a) 3/16
(b) 1/2
(c) 1/4
(d) 2/5

64

Just for practice, subtract the following fractions:

(a) 11/16
   −8/16
   _____

(b) 3/5
   −1/10
   _____

(c) 2/5
   −3/20
   _____

(d) 9/10
   −2/4
   _____

65

gr. 1 3/4

65

The subtraction of mixed numbers may well be easy for you. Let's suppose that you have given a patient gr. 1 3/4 from an ampule that contained gr. iiiss. of a certain drug, and that you must account for the amount left in the ampule. When you subtract the amount given from the amount on hand, you will have a remainder of _____ grain(s).

If your answer to the question in Frame 65 was wrong, and you would like to review the subtraction of mixed numbers, go on to Frame 66. If you are sure that you can do such problems easily, go on to Frame 69.

66

66

fractions

Remember that when we add mixed numbers we add the fractions first. The same rule applies to the subtraction of mixed numbers. Our first step, then, is to subtract the_____in the mixed number.

67

67

whole number

Once again we can see the similarity between mixed numbers and numbers having two digits. When the fraction in the subtrahend (bottom number) is larger than the fraction in the minuend (top number), we "borrow" from the column on the left. In subtracting mixed numbers we sometimes must borrow from the   ·   whole number / fraction column   ·

68

68

Let's say our problem is:

$$4\ 1/3$$
$$-\ 2\ 2/3$$

1 2/3

69

69

We have changed it to:

1 2/3

$$3 \ 4/3$$
$$-2 \ 2/3$$

The answer is: _____

69

(a) 2 9/16
(b) 9 5/8
(c) 1 1/2
(d) 3 3/10

69

Work these subtraction problems for practice:

(a) 4 5/8
    − 2 1/16
    _____

(b) 25 1/8
    − 15 1/2
    _____

(c) 6 1/3
    − 4 5/6
    _____

(d) 5 9/10
    − 2 3/5
    _____

70

$1/2 \times 1/4$

70

It is often necessary for the nurse to multiply fractions as she prepares medications for administration; and the nurse can easily make a serious mistake in dosage if she does not understand exactly what she is doing when she multiplies fractions.

First of all, it is necessary to recognize that 1/2 of 1/4 is a problem in *multiplication*. To find the answer, we would write the problem:

_____ × _____

71

multiply
1/300

71

We have said that the word "of" in a problem involving fractions tells us that we must_____. In a situation in which the nurse must give 1/2 of 1/150, should she administer 1/75 or 1/300 ?
_____.

If you got the right answer to the question in Frame 71, go on to Frame 75. If not, continue with Frame 72 for a fuller explanation.

72

2 × 3

72

Multiplying fractions involves first multiplying the numerators together and then multiplying the denominators together. To multiply 2/3 × 3/4, we would first multiply_____ × _____ to find the product of the numerators.

73

denominators

73

Our next step is to multiply 3 × 4, to find the product of the_____.

74

6/12
1/2

74

After we have found the product of the numerators and the product of the denominators, we reduce the fraction to its lowest terms:
$$2/3 \times 3/4 = \underline{\qquad}$$
(fraction)
This fraction can be reduced to_____.

75

divide
the same

75

To simplify the multiplication of fractions,
we can divide any numerator and denominator by the same number. This is called
"cancellation." When we "cancel," we
_____ any numerator and any denominator by_____ _____number.

76

2

76

Let's simplify the problem $2/3 \times 3/4$ by
cancelling:

$$\frac{2}{3} \times \frac{3}{4}$$

You can see that both 2 and 4 can be
evenly divided by_____.

77

3

77

Now your problem is changed to look like
this:

$$\cdot \; ^1\cancel{2} \atop 3 \times \cancel{4}_2$$

You can also see that the numerator 3
and denominator 3 can both be evenly
divided by_____.

78

1/2

78

Thus, dividing the 3 in the numerator and the 3 in the denominator each by 3, our problem looks like this:

$$\frac{\overset{1}{\cancel{2}}}{\underset{1}{\cancel{3}}} \times \frac{\overset{1}{\cancel{3}}}{\underset{2}{\cancel{4}}} = \frac{1}{1} \times \frac{1}{2}$$

Multiplying this out gives us _____
(fraction)

79

1/6

79

If a patient is to receive 1/2 of an ampule of Pantopon that contains gr. 1/3, you should know that the patient is to receive _____ grain(s).

80

$$\frac{3}{5} \times \frac{14}{1}$$

80

Multiplying fractions by whole numbers really isn't any different from multiplying fractions. All we need to do is write the whole number as the numerator and use 1 as the denominator. To multiply $3/5 \times 14$, we would write our problem like this (supply the missing denominator):

$$\frac{3}{5} \times \frac{14}{\underline{}}$$

81

600

81

If 2/5 of a 1500-calorie diet consists of protein, we can calculate that protein provides_____calories in the diet.

82

8/5
15/4

82

The multiplication of mixed numbers is just as easy if you change the mixed numbers to improper fractions, and then multiply the fractions.

To multiply 1 3/5×3 3/4, you must first change 1 3/5 to_____and 3 3/4 to

_____.

83

5 5/8

83

Now let's see how you would use the multiplication of mixed numbers in a nursing situation. Your instructor adds 1 1/2 ampules of a drug to some intravenous fluid. Each ampule contains 3 3/4 grains of the drug.

Administering 1 1/2 ampules containing 3 3/4 grains each would give the patient a total of_____grain(s) of the drug.

84

5 1/4 quarts

84

Here's another situation: The nurse must prepare a 3 1/2 days' supply of tube feeding for a patient. The daily amount necessary for this patient is 1 1/2 quarts.

The total amount of tube feeding that the nurse should prepare for this patient would be_____quart(s).

85

(a) 1/6
(b) 30/7
(c) 1/75
(d) 75/8

85

For review in multiplying several different types of fractions, work the following problems:

(a) $4/12 \times 3/6$ _____
(b) $15 \times 2/7$ _____
(c) $1/150 \times 2$ _____
(d) $2\ 1/2 \times 3\ 6/8$ _____

$2\ ^{1}/_{8} \times 3\ ^{6}/_{8}$

86

3/4

86

Dividing fractions can be a little tricky, but if you remember the first step the rest is easy. When we divide fractions we must first *invert the divisor*. The divisor is the number you "divide by." If you have 7/8 divided by 3/4, should you invert 7/8 or 3/4?

87

4/3

87

To "invert" means to turn upside down or to reverse positions. When you invert 3/4 it becomes _____.

88

multiplication

88

When you invert the divisor, you reverse the process of division and change it into its exact opposite, which is multiplication. Inverting the fraction you want to divide by changes the problem from one of division to one of _____.

89

89

1/2

Let's say that a nurse must divide 1/6 by 1/3 to determine how much of a fractional dose to give. She must write her problem as $1/6 \div 1/3$. After inverting the divisor and multiplying the fractions, the answer is_____.

90

90

improper
fractions

Dividing mixed numbers presents no problem, because the mixed numbers can be changed to_____fractions. After you have made this change, the problem is simply a matter of dividing the

_____.

91

91

(a) 4/45
(b) 7/2
(c) 152/33
(d) 1/2

Just for practice, work the following problems in division:

    (a) $1/15 \div 3/4$ =_____
    (b) $2/3 \div 4/21$ =_____
    (c) $6\ 1/3 \div 1\ 3/8$=_____
    (d) $1/300 \div 1/150$=_____

POST-TEST ON THE APOTHECARIES' SYSTEM

A. Complete the following table of equivalents:

1. _____minims = 1 dram
2. _____drams = 1 ounce
3. _____ounces = 1 pint
4. _____pints = 1 quart
5. _____ounces = 1 quart
6. _____quarts = 1 gallon

B. Write the correct abbreviations for the following:

1. gallon _____
2. quart _____
3. pint _____
4. ounce _____
5. dram _____
6. grain _____

C. Write the correct symbols for the following:

1. ounce _____
2. dram _____
3. minim _____

D. Write the following dosages as they would be read aloud, that is, "two and one-half drams."

1. ℥ iiss. _____
2. ℥ iv _____
3. ℨ ii _____
4. ℥ ss. _____
5. ℨ viii _____
6. ℳ xiii _____
7. ℳ vii _____
8. gr. viiss _____
9. gr. xx _____
10. gr. xv _____

E. Chart the following dosages using the correct symbols, abbreviations, and numbers:

1. Three ounces of mineral oil: _____
2. One and one-half drams of cascara: _____
3. Fifteen minims of tincture of belladonna: _____
4. One-half dram of Elixir of Donnatal: _____
5. Five grains of aspirin: _____

F. Situations:

1. A solution of 3% aluminum acetate is to be prepared for use as cold compresses. If 2 patients on the ward are receiving the compresses 4 times daily and 8 ounces of solution is needed for each application,_____quart(s) of solution must be prepared for a one-day supply. This is the same as_____gallon(s).
2. Milk of magnesia is a laxative that is used frequently. The nurse on postpartum has 18 patients who are to receive 1 ounce of the medication this p.m. If the stock bottle contains one pint, will there be sufficient medication for all the patients?_____.

3. Mrs. Hamer received Sodium Butisol gr. 1/4 at 10:00 a.m., gr. 3/4 at 2:00 p.m. and gr. ss. at 6:00 p.m. The recommended daily dosage as a sedative should not exceed 2 grains daily. Did she receive more than the usual daily dosage?_____.

4. The physician has ordered ℥ ss. of hydrochloric acid for a patient with pernicious anemia. Before diluting in a larger container, this medication should be measured in a

_____ _____ or _____

_____.

5. What would be the total number of grains received by a patient who is given gr. ss, gr. 1/6, and gr. 3 3/4 of a certain drug?_____.

6. The doctor has ordered Dilaudid gr. 1/64 and the ampule contains gr. 1/32._____ grain(s) of medication will remain in the ampule after the dosage has been withdrawn.

7. Let's suppose that a patient is given gr. 3 3/4 from an ampule containing gr. viiss. The amount left in the ampule will be gr._____.

8. If you were to give a patient 1/2 of a tablet that contains gr. 1/4, how many grains would the patient receive?_____.

9. If you gave a patient 2 tablets containing gr. 1/150 each, would the patient receive a total of gr. 1/300 or gr. 1/75?

_____

10. The patient is to receive Atropine gr. 1/100. If it is available in tablets containing gr. 1/200, you would give the patient _____tablet(s).

PART THREE

THE HOUSEHOLD SYSTEM

1

1

teaspoon
tablespoon

We have said that when drugs are administered in the home it is often necessary to measure them in some household article such as a teaspoon or tablespoon. These articles are not always standard in size, however, and they should be used only if the drug is prescribed according to a unit of measure from the household system.

Two units of measure in the household system are the _____ and _____ .

2

2

4 teaspoonfuls

In the hospital when medications are ordered according to the household system, the nurse should use a medicine glass graduated in household units. Look at the drawing below.

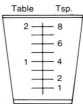

_____teaspoonfuls = 1 tablespoonful

3

2 tablespoonfuls

3

This glass (pictured front and back) is a 1 ounce glass.

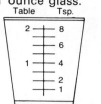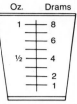

You can see that there are approximately _____ tablespoonfuls in 1 ounce.

4

1 dram

4

Look at the drawing in Frame 3. A teaspoonful is approximately equivalent to what unit of measure in the apothecaries' system?_____.

POST-TEST ON THE HOUSEHOLD SYSTEM

Situations:

1. A clinic patient has been instructed to take 1 tablespoonful of Kaon elixir twice daily. He is receiving the average daily dosage of_____ounce(s) per day.

2. The doctor has ordered 1 teaspoonful of Elixir of Donnatal to be given before each meal and at bedtime. The patient is given a total of_____tablespoonful(s) daily.

3. The order reads Mineral Oil ℥ ss. This could be measured as_____tablespoonful(s).

4. A patient is to receive two teaspoonfuls of Maalox four times each day. The drug is supplied in 12 ounce bottles. How many bottles will she need to take home for a two weeks' supply?_____.

PART FOUR

THE METRIC SYSTEM

UNIT I

REVIEW OF DECIMALS

1

measurement

1

The metric system is the system of
_____ _____ that the nurse will
find most useful, because it is the one most
frequently used in the official listings of
drugs. The metric system is very logically
organized, and it uses decimal numbers for
expressing various amounts. This makes it
necessary to have a full understanding of
decimals before we begin to study the metric
system.

2

10
10

2

The word decimal comes from the Latin
word for "ten." The decimal system is
based on the number 10. A decimal fraction
is a fraction whose denominator is the
number_____ or some power of the
number _____ .

3

denominator
decimal

3

We have said that, besides the number 10
itself, the_____of a _____
fraction can also be a power of 10.
The word "power" in this sense means a
number multiplied by itself a certain number
of times. For example, 10 × 10 × 10 =
1000; and therefore 1000 is known as the
third power of 10.

4

power

4

We can use the decimal system to express mixed numbers or fractions, but the denominator of a decimal fraction must be the number 10 or some_____ of 10, such as 100, 1000, or 10,000.

5

75/100 (Because the denominator is a power of 10.)

5

Which of the following fractions could also be written as a decimal fraction?

2/3   75/100   10/25

6

left
right

6

There are three parts to a decimal: the integer (whole number), the decimal point, and the decimal fraction. Look at their relative positions in the drawing:

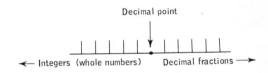

If you wanted to write the mixed number 1 5/10 as a decimal fraction, you would write the whole number 1 to the · left/ right · of the decimal point, and the fraction 5/10 to the · left / right · of the decimal point.

7

decrease

7

The position of a number in relation to the decimal point is called the place value of the number. In the drawing, you can see that decimal fractions · decrease/increase · in value as the number moves farther to the right of the decimal point.

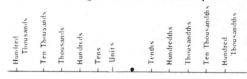

8

increases

8

Just as the decimal fraction has a definite value by virtue of its position, the integer also has a place value—but in exactly the opposite direction. As the whole number moves farther to the left of the decimal point, the value of the integer · increases / decreases ·

9

thousandths

9

The place value or position of a number in relation to the decimal point gives the decimal number its place name.

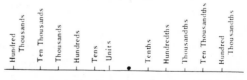

A number in the third position to the right of the decimal point would have the place name_____.

10

thousandths

10

The number 0.365 would therefore be read as "three hundred and sixty-five

_____ .

11

tenths

11

A number in the first position to the right of the decimal point would have the place name _____ .

12

two tenths

12

A decimal written as 0.2 is read as

_____ .

13

eight hundredths

13

A number in the second position to the right of the decimal point would have the place name "hundredths." Thus, 0.08 is read as _____ _____ .

14

0.365

14

To eliminate confusion from overlooking the decimal point and reading a decimal fraction as a whole number, a zero is placed to the left of decimal point when there is no integer in the decimal. Three hundred sixty-five thousandths should be written as _____ .

15

0.75

15

A decimal that reads seventy-five hun‑ dredths should be written as _____ .

16

fourteen and
three hundred
sixty-five
thousandths

16

The number to the left of the decimal point is read just as you would read any whole number. The decimal point itself is read as "and". Thus you would read the figure 14.365 as "_____

_____."

17

one and twenty-
five hundredths

17

A physician's order written as 1.25 mg. of a certain drug should be read as_____

_____ milligrams.

18

are

18

We have said that the decimal fraction takes its value from its position in relation to the decimal point. If this is true, then 0.5 and 0.50 • are/are not • of equal value.

19

value

19

You will recall that reducing a common fraction does not change its value. For instance, 50/100 can be reduced to 5/10 without altering the value of the fraction. Therefore, changing 0.5 to 0.50 does not alter the_____of the decimal fraction.

20

_20_

does not
change

20

If 0.5 and 0.50 are of equal value, then it should be possible to annex zeros to the decimal fraction without changing its value. By "annexing zeros" we mean placing additional zeros to the right of the fraction number. Placing extra zeros to the right of a decimal fraction · changes/does not change · the value of the fraction.

_21_

```
  0.30
+ 0.25
------
  0.55
```

21

This trick of annexing zeros comes in very handy when adding decimals. The numbers to be added are placed so that the decimal points are lined up directly under one another, and then zeros can be annexed when they are needed.

   Show how you would write out the problem 0.3 + 0.25:

```
+ _____
  _____
```
Your answer: _____

_22_

```
  3.500
  0.250
+ 0.001
------
  3.751
```

22

How would you annex zeros to add 3.5, 0.25, and 0.001 ?

```
  _____
  _____
+ _____
```
Your answer: _____

23

decimal points

23

In the subtraction of decimals, we line up the decimal points just as we do for addition. Whenever we subtract decimals, we should annex zeros so that the_____

_____ are directly under one another.

24

$$\begin{array}{r} 2.50 \\ -\,0.08 \\ \hline 2.42 \end{array}$$

24

When we subtract decimals, we write the problem just as we would for whole numbers. The decimal point in the remainder (that is, the answer) is lined up with the decimal points in the minuend and the subtrahend.

Show how you would write out the problem 2.5 − 0.08:

Your answer: _____

25

$$\begin{array}{r} 12.25 \\ -\,7.50 \\ \hline 4.75 \end{array}$$

25

Let's suppose that the nurse in charge must order medication for a patient who is leaving the hospital in the morning. She has in the medicine cabinet 12.25 mg. of the drug, and the patient will receive 7.5 mg. during the night. In order to determine how much of the drug will be left for the patient to take home in the morning, the nurse must subtract 7.5 mg from 12.25 mg. Her answer is _____ mg.

26

decimal point

26

The multiplication of decimals is easy if we remember that the only thing that distinguishes decimal numbers from whole numbers is the decimal point. The multiplication of decimal numbers is done in exactly the same way as the multiplication of whole numbers, except for the placing of the _____ _____ in the product.

27

three

27

After multiplying our decimal numbers, we must determine the proper location of the decimal point in the product. This is done simply by counting the total number of decimal places in the multiplier and the multiplicand. Thus, if there are two decimal places in the multiplier and one decimal place in the multiplicand, there will be a total of _____ decimal places in the product.

28

right

28

When we say decimal places we mean the number of places to the right of the decimal point. If you have a total of three decimal places to account for in the product, then you must have three numbers to the ·
left/right   ·   of the decimal point.

29

Let's suppose that we need to multiply 0.0004 times 0.356. After we have multiplied the numbers, we must place the decimal point so as to have a total of _____ decimal places to the right of the decimal point in the product.

30

To multiply 0.60 × 2.49, we would proceed just as we would for multiplying whole numbers, and then determine the location of the decimal point by counting the total number of decimal places in the multiplier and multiplicand. If our product for 0.60 × 2.49 is 14940, then the decimal point is placed between the _____ and the _____.

31

Sometimes, when we multiply decimals, the product contains fewer figures than we have decimal places. In this case we must prefix as many zeros as necessary. If, for example, the product is 365 and we need five decimal places, we would have to place two _____ in front of the 365.

32

Now our 365 becomes 0.00365 because we have prefixed two zeros in order to have enough decimal places. Prefixing zeros means placing the required number of zeros · in front of/behind · the product.

33

three

33

When we multiply decimals, we know that we must finish with a definite number of decimal places in the product. In the problem 0.2 × 0.03, the product is six thousandths. Therefore we must account for_____ decimal places in the product.

34

two
0.006

34

Since we know that we must account for three decimal places, we prefix_____ zeros to the decimal fraction. The six thousandths is therefore written as the decimal number,_____ .

35

0.000028

35

After multiplying 0.014 × 0.002, we will need six decimal places in the product. The problem would be written:

$$\begin{array}{r} 0.014 \\ \times\,0.002 \\ \hline \end{array}$$

Your answer:_____

36

one

36

The multiplication of a decimal by the number 10 or any multiple of 10 is easy. Each time we move the decimal point one place to the right, we have multiplied by 10. If we wished to multiply 27.3 by 10, we would move the decimal point_____ place(s) to the right.

37

three

37

If we multiply by 10 each time that we move the decimal point one place to the right, then moving the decimal point three places to the right would be the same as 10 × 10 × 10, or 1000 times the number. To multiply 6.3 × 1000, all you need to do is move the decimal point_____ places to the right.

38

two
425

38

Moving the decimal point to the right is a short-cut for multiplying by 10 or any power of 10. A quick way to multiply 4.25 by 100 is to move the decimal point_____ place(s) to the right. The product of 4.25 × 100 is_____ .

39

divisor: 6
dividend: 30
quotient: 5

39

Decimal numbers are divided the same way whole numbers are divided. The only difference is that you must be sure to account for the decimal point. An ordinary problem in division is made up of three parts, which are named as follows:

$$\text{divisor}\,)\overline{\text{dividend}}^{\textstyle\text{quotient}}$$

In the problem 30 ÷ 6, the divisor is _____, and the dividend is_____; the quotient (that is, the answer) would be_____ .

40

0.5

40

In dividing with decimals, it is only necessary to remember to keep the decimal point in the quotient directly above the decimal point in the dividend. Therefore, in the problem 3.5 ÷ 7, the quotient would be_____.

41

whole number

41

One important point to remember in the division of decimals is that the divisor must always be a whole number. In a problem in which the divisor is a decimal number, you must move the decimal point to the right as many places as necessary to change the decimal number into a_____

_____.

42

two
right

42

Whole numbers are always written to the left of the decimal point. To change 0.46 to a whole number, you would move the decimal point_____ places to the

_____.

43

divisor
    (0.46 becomes
    46)
dividend
    (3.22 becomes
    322)

43

Since moving the decimal point changes the place value of a number, we cannot move the decimal point in the divisor without also moving it the same number of places in the dividend. Before we can divide 3.22 by 0.46, we must move the decimal point two places to the right in both the
_____and the_____.

44

right

If we move the decimal point in the divisor we must also move it in the dividend. The decimal point in the quotient is placed above the decimal point in the dividend after it has been moved.

In the problem 3.22 ÷ 0.46, the decimal point is placed to the   •   left/right   •   of the 7 in the quotient.

45

zeros
2500.0

In some problems of division, the dividend is a whole number but the divisor is a decimal number. When the dividend is a whole number, it is understood that the decimal point is located to the right of that number (thus 25 could be read as 25.0).

In a problem in which the divisor is 0.05 and the dividend is 25, we must move the decimal point two places to the right in both the divisor and the dividend. Since there are no numbers to the right of the whole number 25, we must annex two

_____ before we can move the decimal point to the right.

After moving the decimal point in the divisor, 0.05 becomes 05.0 (which is the same as 5); and after moving the decimal point in the dividend, the whole number 25 becomes_____.

500

46

After we have annexed the necessary zeros and moved the decimal points, our problem looks like this:

$$05.) \overline{2500.0}$$

The quotient is_____ .

4

47

To divide 10 by 2.5 we must change our divisor to a whole number, annex zeros to the dividend, and move the decimal point. The problem is written:

$$25.) \overline{100}$$

The quotient is_____.

80

48

Now let's say that we need to divide 280 by 3.5. Move the decimal points and find the quotient. Your answer is_____ .

0.06

49

Sometimes when we divide decimals we find that our divisor is larger than our dividend. When this happens, we can annex as many zeros as we need in the dividend, without moving the decimal point in either the divisor or the dividend.

In the problem 0.3 ÷ 5, we change the 0.3 to 0.30 and divide as we would for whole numbers. Thus, 0.30 ÷ 5 _____ .

50

0.0005

50

Suppose that we had to divide 0.006 by 12. We know that we must annex zeros and divide just as we would for whole numbers, being sure to place the decimal point in the quotient directly above the decimal point in the dividend.

The quotient of 0.006 ÷ 12 is _____.

51

left

51

Dividing is the opposite of multiplying. A short cut for multiplying a number by 10 or powers of 10 is to move the decimal point to the right. A quick and easy way to divide by 10 or powers of 10 is to move the decimal point to the _____.

52

two

52

To divide 10.5 by 100, we can take a short cut and simply move the decimal point _____ places to the left.

53

0.02287

53

The problem 22.87 ÷ 1000 can be easily solved by moving the decimal point to the left. Our answer is _____.

54

0.8

54

A common fraction can easily be changed to a decimal fraction. For instance, 4/5 is the same as 4 ÷ 5. Dividing 4 by 5 is no problem because we can annex as many zeros as necessary to the dividend.

To change 4/5 to a decimal, we write the problem as:

$$5 \overline{)\ 4.0}$$

The answer is _____ .

55

0.6

55

If we needed to change 3/5 to a decimal fraction, we would write our problem as 3 ÷ 5.

The answer is_____ .

56

right

56

Mixed numbers also can be changed to decimals without difficulty. The integer (whole number) is simply written to the left of the decimal point. The common fraction, however, must be changed to a decimal fraction. Decimal fractions are always written to the_____ of the decimal point.

57

12.5

57

The mixed number 12 1/2 contains an integer and a common fraction. This mixed number can be written as the decimal number_____ .

58

3.75

58

If we changed the common fraction in the mixed number 3 3/4 to a decimal fraction, and wrote the mixed number as a decimal, we would have_____ .

59

5/100

59 .   .

To reverse the process and write a decimal fraction as a common fraction, we simply write the fraction as we would read it aloud. For instance, 0.05 is read as "five hundredths." Written as a common fraction, 0.05 would be_____ .

                    fraction

60

33/1000

60

We read 0.033 as thirty-three thousandths. We write it as the common fraction_____ .

61

(a) 1 1/4
(b) 75/10000
(c) 64/100
(d) 0.02
(e) 0.375
(f) 0.05

61

A nurse will encounter many situations in which she must write decimal fractions as common fractions, and in which she must change common fractions to decimal fractions. For practice, work the following problems:

(a)	1.25	=_____	(mixed number)
(b)	0.0075	=_____	(common fraction)
(c)	0.64	=_____	(common fraction)
(d)	1/50	=_____	(decimal fraction)
(e)	3/8	=_____	(decimal fraction)
(f)	1/20	=_____	(decimal fraction)

UNIT II
UNITS OF MEASURE IN THE METRIC SYSTEM

1

secondary

1

Now you should be ready to learn the units of measure in the metric system. These consist of the primary units (the ones on which the system is based) and the secondary units (which are derived from the primary units). In nursing we are chiefly concerned with only two primary units in the metric system: the liter and the gram.

In the metric system, all units of measure derived from the liter and the gram are _____ units.

2

grams

2

The liter is the primary unit used in measuring liquid capacity; the gram is the primary unit used in measuring solid weight. A solid drug would therefore be weighed in

· liters/grams ·

3

measured in liters

3

Because some liquids are much more viscous and therefore heavier than other liquids that might occupy the same amount of space, we usually speak of weighing solids and measuring liquids. You would expect a saline solution to be ·

weighed in grams/measured in liters ·

4

liter

4

We have said that secondary units are derived from primary units. The nomenclature used in medical science contains many terms that are combinations of prefixes or suffixes taken from Latin or Greek. The naming of secondary units is an example of this type of self-explanatory nomenclature.

For example the prefix *milli-* means one-thousandth. The secondary unit called *milliliter* simply means one thousandth of a _____.

5

1000 milliliters

5

If the word milliliter means one-thousandth of a liter, then we know that there are _____ milliliters in 1 liter.

6

milligram

6

The *milliliter* is a secondary unit of measure because it is derived from the primary unit, the liter. By adding the prefix *milli-* to the primary unit *gram*, we have another secondary unit; it is called the

_____.

7

gram

7

There are 1000 milligrams in 1 gram. Another way of expressing this is to say: 1 milligram equals 0.001 _____.

8

liter
gram
milliliter
milligram

8

The prefix *milli-* is used in naming secondary units of measure. Other prefixes may be used, but they are rarely applied in the calculation of dosage. Thus there are really only four units of measure which the nurse will use regularly. These are the primary units: the _____ and the _____ and the secondary units: the _____ and the _____.

UNIT III

ABBREVIATIONS, SYMBOLS, AND NUMBERS IN THE METRIC SYSTEM

1

liter

1

Now we should turn our attention to the abbreviations used for units of measure in the metric system. The abbreviation for liter is simply the first letter of the word; thus L. is the abbreviation for _____

2

ml.

2

The abbreviation for milliliter is the first letter of the prefix *milli-* plus the first letter of the word liter. The abbreviation for milliliter is _____ .

3

the same as

3

Another abbreviation commonly used to designate one-thousandth of a liter is "cc." The cc. abbreviation stands for *cubic centimeter*, which is the amount of space occupied by one milliliter.

Thus 1 cc. is · smaller than/the same as/larger than · 1 milliliter.

4

2

4

The drawing below shows a 2 cc. syringe. This syringe could be used for administering no more than _____ ml. of medication.

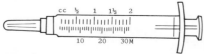

5

metric
secondary
metric

5

The liter and the meter are both primary units of the _____ system; therefore, the milliliter and centimeter are both _____ units of the _____ system.

6

grams

6

The abbreviation for gram is Gm. We use a capital G to avoid confusing Gm. with gr., the abbreviation for grain. A dosage of 0.1 Gm. means that the drug has been weighed and dispensed in   •   grains/grams   •

7

mg.

7

The abbreviation for milliliter is a combination of the first letter of the prefix *milli-* and the first letter of the word *liter*. The abbreviation for milligram is formed from a similar combination. The abbreviation for milligram is _____ .

8

0.25 mg.

8

We have said that the metric system is based on the decimal system. Thus, only decimals are used to designate amounts in the metric system. The decimal number is always written before an abbreviation for a unit of measure. Twenty-five hundredths of a milligram should be written as _____ .

9

If a physician orders one-tenth milligram of digitoxin, how would you chart the dosage, using the proper abbreviation and decimal numbers? _____ .

Did you remember to place a zero in front of the decimal point, to prevent errors in reading?

10

Sometimes we administer one and one-half milliliters by injection. This amount should be written as _____ .

11

The dosage on a medicine card is written aspirin 0.3 Gm. You would read this as three-tenths of a _____ .

12

We have said that milliliters and cubic centimeters both express one-thousandth of a liter. Suppose that you were going to give a patient 0.5 ml. of a drug, and that your syringe was graduated in cc's. You would pull the plunger up to the line marked
•   1/2 cc. / 2 cc. / 5 cc.   •

UNIT IV
EXCHANGING WEIGHTS WITHIN THE METRIC SYSTEM

1

1000 milligrams

1

Sometimes drugs are weighed and dispensed from the hospital pharmacy in grams, when the dosage is ordered in milligrams. In this instance the nurse must be able to change the milligrams into grams.

Let's say that we have 2000 milligrams. We know that if 1000 milligrams are equal to 1 gram, then 2000 milligrams will be equal to 2 grams.

In changing the milligrams to grams, we divide the number of milligrams by 1000 because there are_____ milligrams in each gram.

2

three
left

2

There is an easy way to divide by 1000 when changing milligrams to grams. You will recall that if you wish to divide by 1000 you can simply move the decimal point three places to the left.

Now you can complete the following rule for changing milligrams to grams: To change milligrams to grams, move the decimal point_____places to the

_____.

3

(a) 2 Gm.
(b) 0.5 Gm
(c) 0.25 Gm
(d) 0.1 Gm.

3

Change the following milligrams to grams:

(a) 2000 mg. = _____ Gm.
(b) 500 mg. = _____ Gm.
(c) 250 mg. = _____ Gm.
(d) 100 mg. = _____ Gm.

4

0.5 Gm.

4

Now you are ready to solve some problems of the kind that may confront a nurse as she prepares to give medications.

Suppose that the physician orders 500 mg. of a certain drug and that the drug is dispensed in 0.5 Gm. tablets. By moving the decimal point, you could determine that 500 mg. are equal to_____ Gm.

5

1 tablet

5

Since 500 mg. are equal to 0.5 Gm., this patient should receive_____ tablet(s).

6

3 tablets

6

Let's say that a dose of 750 mg. of a certain drug has been ordered, and that the drug is dispensed in scored tablets of 0.25 Gm. each. The patient should be given_____ tablet(s).

7

1/4 tablet

7

Let's say that a physician orders 250 mg. of a medication that is dispensed in scored tablets of 1 Gm. each. The patient should receive_____ tablet(s).

8

8

scored

8

In Frame 7 the patient was given 1/4 of a tablet. This was done using a scored tablet; that is one with grooves in it allowing for accurate fractional doses. Tablets that are grooved so that they can be broken into accurate halves or fourths are called _____ tablets.

9

100 mg.
2 tablets

9

Swallowing large numbers of tablets or capsules is difficult for some persons. To avoid unnecessary discomfort for her patient the nurse should choose, from available drugs of varying strengths, the tablet or capsule that contains the amount most nearly equivalent to the dosage ordered for the patient.

If, for example, a patient is to receive 0.2 Gm. of a drug and there are available tablets of 10, 50, and 100 mg. each, which strength tablet would be most appropriate? _____ . How many would you give? _____ .

10

2 capsules

10

If a physician orders 4 mg. of a drug, and the label on the container reads 0.002 Gm. per capsule, the nurse should give the patient _____ capsule(s).

11

0.1 Gm.
1 capsule

11

When a nurse prepares to give 100 mg. of Seconal, she finds that the drug is dispensed in 0.1 Gm. capsules. Since 100 mg. equals _____ Gm., the nurse would give _____ capsule(s).

12

cannot

12

We have said that scored tablets can be divided to give accurate fractional doses. Capsules, on the other hand, are never scored for divided doses. The nurse. can/cannot · administer less than one capsule.

13

three
right

13

It is only logical to recognize that if we can change milligrams to grams by moving the decimal point three places to the left, we can change the grams back to milligrams by moving the decimal point_____ places to the_____

14

three
right

14

Let's see if you can complete a rule tor changing grams to milligrams: To change grams to milligrams, move the decimal point_____places to the _____.

(a) 100 mg.
(b) 340 mg.
(c) 2 mg.
(d) 250 mg.
(e) 15 mg.

15

Work the following problems according to the rule that you have written:

(a)	0.1 Gm.	= _____	mg.
(b)	0.34 Gm.	= _____	mg.
(c)	0.0020 Gm.	= _____	mg.
(d)	0.25 Gm.	= _____	mg.
(e)	0.015 Gm.	= _____	mg.

16

500 mg.

2 capsules

16

The physician orders 0.5 Gm. of Panalba, and the label on the bottle reads 250 mg. per capsule. Since 0.5 Gm. is equal to _____ mg., the nurse should give the patient _____ capsule(s).

17

4 tablets

17

Let's say that a physician orders 2 Gm. of Gantrisin as a "stat" dose and that the medication is dispensed in 500-mg. tablets. How many tablets should the patient receive? _____ .

18

(a) 500 mg.
(b) 5 mg.
(c) 0.03 Gm.
(d) 0.015 Gm.
(e) 0.004 Gm.
(f) 0.4 mg.
(g) 0.75 Gm.
(h) 600 mg.
(i) 0.3 Gm.
(j) 0.12 Gm.

18

To test your ability to change milligrams to grams, and grams to milligrams, complete the following table:

(a)	0.5 Gm.	_____ mg.
(b)	0.005 Gm.	_____ mg.
(c)	30 mg.	_____ Gm.
(d)	15 mg.	_____ Gm.
(e)	4 mg.	_____ Gm.
(f)	0.0004 Gm.	_____ mg.
(g)	750 mg.	_____ Gm.
(h)	0.6 Gm.	_____ mg.
(i)	300 mg.	_____ Gm.
(j)	120 mg.	_____ Gm.

POST-TEST ON THE METRIC SYSTEM

A. Complete the following table of equivalents:

1. _____ml. = 1 liter
2. _____cc. = 1 ml.
3. _____mg. = 1 gram

B. Write the correct abbreviations for the following:

1. Liter _____
2. Gram _____
3. Milliliter _____
4. Milligram _____
5. Cubic centimeter _____

C. Write the following amounts as they would be read aloud:

1. 0.35 mg. _____
2. 0.2 mg. _____
3. 1.75 mg. _____
4. 0.5 Gm. _____
5. 0.6 ml. _____
6. 0.55 L. _____
7. 2.5 ml. _____
8. 0.04 mg. _____
9. 4.8 L. _____
10. 7.5 Gm. _____

D. Chart the following dosages, using the correct abbreviations and numbers:

1. One and one-half grams _____
2. Three-tenths milligram _____
3. Seven-hundredths milliliter _____
4. Three-fourths liter _____
5. Two and one-half milligrams _____

E. Situations:

1. A physician wishes to replace 2 liters of fluid lost by vomiting and diarrhea. If a bottle of intravenous fluids contains 1000 ml., how many bottles should the patient receive to replace the fluids lost? _____.

2. You must give a patient 0.015 Gm. of a certain drug, and the drug is dispensed in tablets of 5 mg. each. How many tablets would you give him? _____.

3. The proposed daily dosage for metaxalone is 2.4 Gm. The drug is available in 400 mg. tablets. How many tablets would be needed for a one-day supply? _____

4. Suppose that a physician orders 100 mg. of a certain drug and the label on the bottle reads 0.1 Gm. per tablet. How many tablets would the patient receive? _____

5. A child on pediatrics is given a 2.5 ml. dropperful of Erythrocin drops four times daily. He is receiving _____ cc. medication daily. If each 2.5 ml. contains 100 mg. of medication, he receives _____ Gm. of the drug daily.

6. A certain medication is available in 400 mg. tablets and a physician orders 2 Gm. per day. How many tablets would the patient receive each day? _____

7. Mrs. Jamison is to receive 500 mg. of Thiosulfil Forte four times a day for treatment of cystitis. The only tablets available are scored tablets labeled 0.25 Gm. To supply the dosage of 500 mg. the patient should receive _____ tablet(s).

8. An elderly patient with prostatic cancer is to receive 1.25 mg. of Premarin three times daily. Because of difficulty in swallowing, he is receiving the liquid preparation. If 4 cc. contain 0.625 mg. he should receive _____ cc. for each dose. The liquid is supplied in 4-ounce (120 cc.) bottles. This would be sufficient for _____ day(s).

9. Tybamate is a major tranquilizer. The physician has ordered 0.25 Gm. every four hours and you have available capsules containing 125 mg. each. How many capsules should the patient receive every four hours? _____

10. The doctor has ordered 0.2 Gm. of Mebaral. You have available tablets of 32, 50, 100, and 200 mg. each. Which strength would be most appropriate to give and how many tablets would you give? _____

PART FIVE

**EXCHANGING UNITS OF
WEIGHT AND MEASURE
BETWEEN THE
APOTHECARIES' AND THE
METRIC SYSTEMS**

UNIT I

EXCHANGING UNITS OF MEASURE

1

metric

1

When a nurse prepares to give a medication to a patient, she often finds that a physician has ordered the drug in a unit of measure from the apothecaries' system, but that the drug has been prepared and is dispensed in a unit of measure from the metric system.

In this situation the nurse must know both systems so that she can take the unit of measure from the apothecaries' system and find its approximate equivalent in the _____system.

2

conversion

2

When the nurse takes an order in one system and finds its approximate equivalent in another system, she is *converting*. The exchanging of units of weight and measure from one system to another is called

_____.

3

cannot

3

In converting we find *approximately* the same weight or measure in a different system. We • can/cannot • say that the measurements are exactly the same.

4

1000 ml

4

Let's consider how a nurse would use conversion in preparing large amounts of solutions for various treatments.

You will recall that there are 1000 ml. in 1 liter. A quart in the apothecaries' system is equal to approximately 1 liter in the metric system. Therefore, there are approximately _____ ml. in 1 quart.

5

1 liter

5

Suppose that a physician orders 1 quart of soapsuds solution to be given as an enema, but that the only available container is a vessel graduated in liters. In measuring 1 quart of soapsuds solution in this container, the nurse would prepare_____ liter(s).

6

500 cc.

6

There are 2 pints in 1 quart. Since a milliliter is the same amount as a cubic centimeter, you would calculate that there are approximately_____ cc. in 1 pint.

7

1 gallon

7

Let's say you must prepare a one-day supply of boric acid solution to be used for compresses. There are 8 patients receiving these compresses, and each patient will need 500 ml. You know that you must prepare _____ gallon(s) of boric acid solution.

If you worked that problem in Frame 7 correctly, go on to Frame 11. If you did not understand how to solve this problem, go on to Frame 8.

8

4000 ml.

Your first step in solving the problem would be to determine the total number of milliliters needed. Eight patients using 500 ml. each would require a total of_____ml.

9

4 quarts

You would need 4000 ml. of the boric acid solution. If 1000 ml. equal approximately 1 quart, then 4000 ml. would be approximately the same as_____quart(s).

10

1 gallon

Since there are 4 quarts in 1 gallon, and 4000 ml. are equal to 4 quarts, the amount needed for the boric acid compresses would be_____gallon(s).

11

1/2 gallon

In another situation, the nurse must prepare a supply of solution for 10 irrigations. She will need 200 ml. for each irrigation. The total amount of solution needed would be_____gallon(s).

60 ml. (or cc.)

12

Sometimes it is necessary to convert ounces to milliliters. One ounce is equal to approximately 30 ml. A patient receiving milk and cream ℥ ii every hour would be given _____ ml. (or cc.) every hour.

45 ml. (cc.)

13

If a physician orders a dose of ℥ iss. of a certain medication, the nurse could measure this in milliliters. She would give _____ ml. (cc.) of the medication to the patient.

240 cc.

14

If you were measuring and recording a patient's fluid intake in cubic centimeters, how many cc. would you record after a patient drinks an eight-ounces glass of water? _____ .

15 ml.

15

Sometimes a physician will order Gelusil ℥ ss. The nurse would give the patient _____ ml.

16

Suppose that a physician orders 4 cc. of elixir of phenobarbital every 4 hours for 30 doses, and you need to know how many fluid ounces to order from the pharmacy in order to have a sufficient amount of medication on hand.

120 cc. 4 oz.   Four cubic centimeters for 30 doses would be a total of_____cc., or_____ ounce(s).

17

8 oz.

17

If a physician orders 12 cc. of a certain medication to be given 4 times a day for 20 doses, you must order a total of_____ fluid ounces from the pharmacy.

18

4 cc.

18

One dram in the apothecaries' system is equal to approximately 4 ml. in the metric system. If this is true, then 1 dram would contain approximately_____cc.

19

8 ml.

19

If a physician orders ℥ ii of a medication, this would be approximately equivalent to _____ml.

20

(a) 1 dr.
(b) 3 dr.
(c) 4 dr.
(d) 2 1/2 dr.

20

Just for practice, write the equivalents of the following amounts:

(a) 4 ml. _____dr.
(b) 12 ml. _____dr.
(c) 16 ml. _____dr.
(d) 10 ml. _____dr.

21

30 minims

21

It is often necessary to convert milliliters (or cubic centimeters) to minims, especially when preparing solutions to be given by injection. Therefore, it is important to remember that 1 ml. is equal to approximately 15 minims.

A 2-cc. syringe contains _____ minims.

22

10 minims

22

Let's say that you have dissolved a hypodermic tablet in 1 ml. of sterile water, and have calculated that you must give the patient only 2/3 of this amount. The patient will receive _____ minims of the solution.

23

75 mg.

23

Suppose that you have taken a 2-cc. ampule of Demerol from a container labeled 50 mg. per cc. If you gave a patient 22.5 minims, he would receive _____ mg. of the drug.

If you calculated the answer to the problem in Frame 23 correctly, go on to Frame 26. If you would like to see how this problem is solved, go on to Frame 24.

24

15 minims

24

To solve the problem, we must first realize that 50 mg. per cc. is the same as 50 mg. per 15 minims, because there are approximately _____ minims in 1 cc.

25

75 mg.

25

The patient received 22.5 minims, or 1.5 cc. If 1 cc. contains 50 mg., then 1.5 cc. would contain_____ mg.

26

10

26

Let's suppose that you have a 5-cc. vial of a drug and that the patient is to receive 7.5 minims daily. By dividing the total number of minims by the number of minims in each dose, you can determine the total number of doses in the vial. A 5-cc. vial of the drug will provide a patient with_____ daily doses of 7.5 minims each.

27

(a) 1 qt. = 1 L.
(b) 1 qt. =
     1000 ml.
(c) 1 pt. =
     500 ml.
(d) 1 oz. =
     30 ml.
(e) 1 dr. = 4 ml.
(f) 15 minims =
     1 ml.

27

In the process of converting, a nurse must exchange measures in one system into approximate equivalents in another system. Test yourself and see how well you have learned the more commonly used equivalents.

	Apothecaries'	Metric
(a)	1 quart	=_____liter(s)
(b)	1 quart	=_____ml.
(c)	1 pint	=_____ml.
(d)	1 ounce	=_____ml.
(e)	1 dram	=_____ml.
(f)	15 minims	=_____ml.

UNIT II

EXCHANGING UNITS OF WEIGHT

1

proportion

1

Up to this point all the units we have used for conversion have been units of liquid measure. Now we are ready to convert units of weight. The simplest and most practical method for doing this is by using ratio and proportion. This method will stand you in good stead in computation of dosage, too, and does not involve memorizing rules and formulas.

When confronted with the task of exchanging units of weight from one system of measure for another, the nurse need not recall an extensive list of rules and formulas; she can use the simple method of ratio and _____.

2

1 and 15

2

You will remember that a ratio indicates the relationship between two quantities or two numbers. If you write 1:15, you are showing the relationship between _____ and_____.

3

**1,
15**

3

Setting up a ratio is simply a way of making a comparison between two quantities or numbers. The ratio of 1:15 means that one part of a given substance or thing is being compared to 15 parts of another substance or thing. An accepted equivalent for grains and grams is 1 Gm. = 15 gr. The ratio of 1 Gm. : 15 gr. means that_____gram is comparable or equal to_____grains.

4

ratio

4

We can see, then, that the accepted equivalent of 1 Gm. = 15 gr. can be written as the ratio 1 Gm. : 15 gr. When a nurse uses an accepted equivalent from a table of equivalents, she can always express the equivalent as a_____.

5

Gm.,
gr.

5

In converting from one system to another it is very important to label the terms in a ratio. For example, 1:15 tells you nothing about the units of measure being represented. You must write the equivalent 1 Gram is equal to 15 grains as 1_____:15_____.

6

1/15

6

A ratio may be written as a fraction. The first term in the ratio is the numerator of the fraction and the second term is the denominator. The ratio 1 : 15 can be written _____ .

(fraction)

7

the same value as

7

Since a ratio can be written as a common fraction, we can multiply or divide both terms of a ratio by the same number, just as we can multiply or divide both terms of a common fraction by the same number. This does not alter the value of the fraction or the ratio.

The ratio 2 Gm. : 30 gr   •   has the same value as/twice the value of   •   the ratio 1 Gm. : 15 gr.

8

30 grains

8

A proportion shows equality between two ratios. We know that the ratio 1 Gm. : 15 gr. is the same as, or equal to, the ratio 2 Gm.: 30 gr. To express this equality, we write the proportion as 1 Gm. : 15 gr. = 2 Gm. : 30 gr. We can read this proportion to mean that 1 Gm. is comparable to 15 gr. in the same way that 2 Gm. are comparable to _____ .

9

2 Gm. : 30 gr.

9

A proportion is a quick way of showing the similarity between numbers or quantities. If we say "1 gram is similar to 15 grains in the same way that 2 grams are similar to 30 grains," we can see that the equality is expressed in the proportion: 1 Gm. : 15 gr. = _____ Gm.: _____ gr.

10

1 and 30
15 and 2

10

Each of the four parts of a proportion is called a term. The first and fourth are called the extremes; the second and third are called the means. In the proportion 1 Gm.: 15 gr. = 2 Gm. : 30 gr., the *extremes* are the numbers _____ and _____. The *means* are the numbers _____ and _____.

11

multiply

11

In a proportion the product of the means must always equal the product of the extremes. (In mathematics the word product indicates the result of multiplication.) To determine the product of the means and the product of the extremes, we must _____ 2 by 15 and 1 by 30.

12

extremes
means
(either order)

12

Now our proportion of 1 Gm. : 15 gr. = 2 Gm. : 30 gr. becomes 30 = 30. A true proportion must always show that the product of the _____ is equal to the product of the _____.

13

X

When one term of a proportion is not known, it is possible to find the value of this term. First we write our proportion and substitute X for the unknown term. Let's say that we have 1 Gm. : 15 gr. = X Gm. : 3 gr. This proportion means that 1 gram is similar to 15 grains in the same way that _____number of grams is similar to 3 grains.

14

1 × 3 = 3

The proportion is 1 Gm. : 15 gr. = X Gm. : 3 gr. When we multiply the means we have 15 times X or 15X. When we multiply the extremes we have_____ × _____ which equals _____.

15

X = 0.2 Gm.

Setting the product of the means equal to the product of the extremes, we have 15X = 3. We can determine the value of X by dividing 3 by 15. The value of X is _____.

16

left

These are the steps we have taken:

    1 Gm. : 15 gr. = X Gm. : 3 gr.

          15X = 3 (or 3 ÷ 15)

            X = 0.2 Gm.

    In the second step of evaluating X, the X must always be placed to the • left/ right • of the equal sign.

17

3

3

A quick way to prove that your calculation of X is correct is to check to see whether the product of the means does indeed equal the product of the extremes. If you calculated X as 0.2 Gm. in the proportion 1 Gm. : 15 gr. = X Gm. : 3 gr., you could determine that 15 × 0.2 = _____ and that 1 × 3 = _____ .

18

grams to
grains

By now you must surely know that 1 gram is the approximate equivalent of 15 grains. Using this equivalent, try using ratio and proportion for some nursing problems involving converting grams to grains. Remember that in a proportion you must be careful that the units of measure are compared in the same order. If we compare grams to grains in the first ratio we must compare · grains to grams/grams to grains · in the second ratio.

19

gr. 7 1/2

We'll set up the first proportion for you.
1 Gm. : 15 gr. = 0.5 Gm. : X gr.

$$1 X = 15 \times 0.5$$
$$X = \underline{\hspace{1cm}} gr.$$

20

11 1/4 gr.
60 gr.
3 gr.
3 3/4 gr.

20

Here are some more for practice:

0.75 Gm._____gr.
4   Gm._____gr.
0.2   Gm._____gr.
0.25 Gm._____gr.

21

grains to grams

21

Now we will suppose that the physician has ordered a drug in grains and it is dispensed in grams. Whenever a nurse uses conversion it is easier for her if she converts the unit of measure ordered to the unit of measure on hand. Since a nurse must give medication from the units of measure she has available, it is more convenient if in the above situation she will convert   ·
grains to grams/grams to grains   ·

22

3.75 gr.

22

A nurse needs to convert gr. 3 3/4 to grams. Since the dosage on hand is measured in the metric system, and decimal numbers are used, the mixed number 3 3/4 should be changed to a decimal number. When setting up her proportion she should write gr. 3 3/4 as_____.

23

23

0.25 Gm.

Now she has the proportion:
1 Gm. : 15 gr. = X Gm. : 3.75 gr.
$$15X = 3.75$$
$$X = \underline{\hspace{2cm}}$$

24

24

0.1 Gm.

Let's say that a physician orders Nembutal gr. iss, and that the drug is available in capsules labeled 0.1 Gm. each. Using ratio and proportion you will find that gr. iss is equal to_____Gm.

25

25

1 capsule

If the capsules are labeled 0.1 Gm. each and the physician has ordered gr. iss, it is obvious that the patient should receive_____ capsule(s).

26

26

Here are some practice problems:

0.8 Gm.   12   gr._____Gm.
0.3 Gm.   5   gr._____Gm.
3   Gm.   45   gr. _____Gm.
0.05 Gm.   3/4 gr._____Gm.

27

milligrams

27

In the above problems you have exchanged grains and grams using the equivalent 1 Gm. = 15 gr. If you needed to exchange milligrams and grains you should use the equivalent 60 mg. = 1 gr. This can serve as your first ratio when converting _____ to grains.

28

30 mg. : X gr.

28

If, for instance, you needed to convert 30 mg. to an unknown number of grains, your proportion would be 60 mg. : 1 gr. = _____ : _____ .

29

60 mg. : 1 gr.
   = X mg. : 2 gr.

29

Suppose that a physician orders 2 grains of a certain drug and that the dosage on hand is 60-mg. tablets. The first ratio is the conversion factor, 60 mg. = 1 grain. The proportion for converting is:

_____ : _____ = _____ : _____

30

2 tablets

30

When you calculate the value of X, you find that the physician's order of 2 grains can be converted to 120 mg. If 1 tablet of the drug contains 60 mg., then _____ tablet(s) would contain 120 mg.

31

0.4 mg.

31

Suppose that a physician orders atropine gr. 1/150 and that the label on the bottle reads 0.2 mg. per tablet. You must know how many tablets to give the patient, but first you must convert the grains to milligrams.

After setting up your proportion and calculating X, you find that gr. 1/150 is equivalent to _____ mg.

32

2 tablets

32

Your problem was to determine how many tablets to give. You can again find the answer by using ratio and proportion:

0.2 mg. : 1 tablet = 0.4 mg. : X tablets

X = _____ tablet(s)

33

60 mg.: 1 gr. =
X mg.: 1/200 gr.

33

Suppose that a physician orders gr. 1/200 of scopolamine and that the drug is dispensed in 0.3-mg. tablets.

The proportion for converting the order into the dosage on hand is:

_____ : _____ = _____ : _____

34

1 tablet

34

When you calculate the value of X in this proportion, you find that 0.3 mg. is the equivalent of gr. 1/200. Now you know that the physician's order is the same as 0.3 mg. and that the patient should be given_____ tablet(s).

35

35

30 mg.

Suppose that a physician orders codeine gr. ss., and that the drug is dispensed in tablets of 15 mg. each.

After setting up your proportion and calculating the value of X, you find that gr. ss. is equivalent to approximately _____ mg.

36

36

2 tablets

Since you have found that the physician's order of gr. ss. is equivalent to approximately 30 mg., and since the drug is dispensed in tablets of 15 mg. each, you know that the patient should receive_____ tablet(s).

37

37

3/4 tablet

A physician orders gr. 1/4 of a certain drug, and the drug is dispensed in 20-mg. scored tablets. By using the ratio and proportion method, the nurse can determine that the patient should receive _____ tablet(s).

38

38

gr. 1/20
1 tablet

In another situation, you find that a physician has ordered 3 mg. of a certain drug and that the dosage on hand is in gr. 1/20 tablets.

When you calculate the value of X, you find that 3 mg. are equal to_____ grain(s); therefore the patient should receive_____ tablet(s).

39

In working all the problems in this section you have used the equivalents 1 Gm. = 15 gr. and 60 mg. = 1 gr. These equivalents can be found in any table of accepted equivalents. Such a table usually is readily available to the nurse giving medications in a hospital and should be used to avoid confusion and inaccuracy in calculation of dosage.

When a drug is ordered in one system and the dosage on hand is measured in another system, the safest and most accurate way to convert the dosage is by consulting a(n)_____of accepted equivalents.

40

When the dosage ordered is not included in the table of equivalents, or a table is not available, the nurse then uses the equivalents she knows and employs ratio and proportion to compute the dosage.

Two equivalents that you should be thoroughly familiar with at this point are 1 Gm. = _____ gr. and_____mg. = 1 gr.

POST-TEST ON EXCHANGING UNITS
OF WEIGHT AND MEASURE

A. Complete the following table of equivalents:

1. 2 quarts   = _____ liters
2. 1 gallon   = _____ liters
3. 1/2 gallon   = _____ ml.
4. 1000 ml.   = _____ pints
5. 1 ounce   = _____ ml.
6. 8 ml.   = _____ drams
7. 2 ml.   = _____ minims
8. 2/3 ml.   = _____ minims
9. 20 minims   = _____ ml.
10. 1/2 dram   = _____ ml.
11. gr. 1/3   = _____ Gm.
12. gr. 7 1/2   = _____ Gm.
13. 0.25 Gm.   = _____ grains
14. 2 Gm.   = _____ grains
15. 0.2 Gm.   = _____ grains

B. Situations:

1. Wet dressings of potassium permanganate 1:25,000 are to be applied 4 times daily. If 8 ounces of solution is necessary for each application,_____ L. will be needed for a 2-day supply.

2. An infant with anemia is given 20 minims of Feosol

Elixir 3 times daily. This is a total of_____ml. each day. If each 2 drams supplies 5 grains of medication, the infant is receiving_____gr. daily.

3. A patient has been given 0.2 Gm. of a certain drug. This is approximately equivalent to_____gr.

4. The doctor has ordered gr. vi. The tablets on hand are labeled 0.2 Gm. You should give_____tablet(s).

5. A preoperative patient is receiving 180 grains of sulfasuxidine in 4 evenly divided doses. If each tablet contains 0.5 Gm., the patient is given_____tablet(s) for each dose.

6. A physician orders gr. 1/6 of a certain drug. The dosage on hand is in 10-mg. tablets. The patient would receive _____tablet(s).

7. The dosage desired is gr. 1/150. The drug on hand is in tablets of 0.2 mg. each. How many tablets would the patient receive?_____.

8. The dosage desired is gr. 3/4. The drug on hand is in scored tablets of 15 mg. each. How many tablets would the patient receive?_____.

9. A physician orders gr. 1/15 of a drug, and it is available only in 2-mg. tablets. You would give the patient_____ tablet(s).

10. The dosage desired is gr. 1/240 and the drug on hand is in 0.5-mg. scored tablets. The patient would receive _____tablet(s).

PART SIX

PREPARING SOLUTIONS
FOR PARENTERAL
ADMINISTRATION

UNIT I
POWDERED DRUGS

1

diluent

1

Some drugs, such as streptomycin and all-purpose bicillin, are dispensed in powdered or crystalline form. A liquid such as sterile water or saline must be added to dilute these solid drugs before they can be given by injection. This diluting liquid is called a diluent.

The liquid used to dissolve or dilute a powdered drug is called a(n)

_____ .

2

more than
one dose

2

Many solid drugs are dispensed in single-dose vials, but some vials contain enough for several doses. With either the single-dose vial or the multiple-dose vial, a diluent must be added before the drug can be given. A multiple-dose vial contains ·
a single dose / more than one dose ·

3

instructions

3

Most injectable powdered drugs are accompanied by printed instructions provided by the manufacturer and packaged with each vial. When a nurse prepares a powdered drug for injection, she must read the accompanying literature for specific _____ for dissolving the drug.

4

diluent

4

These instructions should tell the nurse exactly how much diluent to use. The small circular accompanying most powdered drugs tells the nurse how much _____ should be used to obtain the desired dosage.

5

0.5 ml.

5

For example, instructions for preparing all-purpose bicillin direct the nurse to reconstitute the sterile dry powder by adding 1.5 ml. of sterile water. This provides a single dose of 2 ml. Since the nurse added only 1.5 ml. of diluent, the volume of the dry drug would account for_____ ml. of finished solution.

6

displacement

6

Frame 5 gives an example of displacement. When drugs increase the volume of solution, the nurse must read the manufacturer's directions, which will have taken into consideration the amount of _____ by the powdered drug after it has been dissolved.

7

2 ml.

7

Let's suppose that a nurse must give 1 Gm. of Staphcillin. She has available a 6.0 Gm. vial with directions as follows: *Add 8.6 ml. of diluent (each ml. will contain 500 mg. Staphcillin).* After adding the diluent as directed the nurse should administer _____ml. of the solution.

8

2.2 ml.

8

In another nursing situation the patient is to receive 0.5 Gm. of Keflin. Directions accompanying the drug read as follows: *Each Gm. should be diluted with 4 ml. of sterile water for injection. This will provide 0.5 Gm. doses of 2.2 ml. each.*

After adding the diluent as directed the nurse will withdraw_____ml. of solution into the syringe in order to give the prescribed dose.

If you answered 2 ml. instead of 2.2 ml., you forgot about the powdered drug adding volume to the solution. Go back and read Frames 5 and 6.

9

diluent

9

When there are no directions accompanying powdered injectable drugs and the nurse has no way of knowing how much volume the dry drug will add to the finished solution, she should consult a pharmacist for assistance in determining the amount of _____ to be added for a proper dosage.

UNIT II

HYPODERMIC TABLETS

1

1 ml.

1

Hypodermic tablets are quite small and can easily be dissolved in sterile water or saline. The average amount of solution given by hypodermic injection is 1 ml.

When dissolving hypodermic tablets, the correct dosage of the drug will usually be dissolved in_____ of diluent.

2

3 ml.

2

Let's say that a physician orders atropine gr. 1/300, and that the dosage is available only in hypodermic tablets of gr. 1/100 each. If each milliliter of the solution is to contain gr. 1/300, the nurse should dissolve the tablet in_____ ml. of sterile water.

If you answered the question in Frame 2 correctly, go on to Frame 6. If you missed this question, go on to Frame 3.

3

1/300 gr.:1 ml.

3

Let's stop and review the information given. First, we know that every 1 ml. of finished solution should contain gr. 1/300, because that is the amount of drug ordered by the physician, and the average amount of solution given hypodermically is 1 ml. Now you set up your first ratio as:

_____ gr. :_____ml.

4

1/100 gr. : X ml.

4

When you set up the second ratio, you find that you do not know the number of milliliters to use as a diluent. You do know, however, the number of grains in each tablet on hand: each tablet contains 1/100 grains. The second ratio is written:

_____ gr. : _____ ml.

5

3 ml.

5

Now you have:

1/300 gr. : 1 ml. = 1/100 gr. : X ml.

When you solve this for X, you find that the tablet should be dissolved in _____ ml. of diluent.

6

gr. 1/300

6

If you dissolve gr. 1/100 in 3 ml. and give a 1 ml. injection, you are giving the patient 1/3 of gr. 1/100, which equals _____ grain(s) of the drug. (fraction)

7

1.5 ml.
0.5 ml.

7

Suppose that a physician orders gr. 1/150 and the drug is dispensed in tablets of 1/100 grains each. If 1 ml. is to contain gr. 1/150, the nurse should dissolve 1 tablet of gr. 1/100 in _____ ml. of diluent and discard _____ ml. of finished solution.

8

8

2 or more

Sometimes the dosage ordered by a physician is larger than the amount contained in a single hypodermic tablet. When the nurse converts the order into the dosage on hand and finds that 1 tablet is not sufficient, she must use_____or more tablets, depending on the amount of drug needed.

9

9

3 tablets
90 mg.

It is easy to determine the number of tablets needed if we simply look at the dosage ordered and the amount on hand. For example, we cannot obtain 45 mg. of a drug from a single 30-mg. tablet. Therefore we must take the dosage from 2 tablets, or 60 mg.

If we need 75 mg. of a drug, and we have on hand only 30-mg. tablets, it will be necessary to use_____tablet(s), which add up to_____mg.

10

10

18

3

15

Your problem is to give 75 mg. in 1 ml. (15 minims). You have 90 mg. on hand (3 30-mg. tablets). To give the patient 75 mg. of the drug you should dissolve the 3 tablets in_____minims of diluent, discard_____minims and give the patient_____minims.

11

11

60 mg.

Suppose that you are instructed to give 50 mg. of a drug hypodermically, and the drug is available in 30 mg. tablets. To obtain 50 mg. in 15 minims of finished solution, you must use 2 tablets of 30 mg. each. Your proportion would be:

50 mg. : 15 minims = _____ mg. : X minims

12

12

18 minims
 3 minims
15 minims

Your proportion is:

50 mg. : 15 minims = 60 mg. : X minims.

   If 15 minims is to contain 50 mg. of the drug, you must dissolve 2 of the 30-mg. tablets in _____ minims of diluent, discard _____ m. and give the patient _____ m.

13

13

2 tablets
20 minims

Suppose that another physician's order reads scopolamine gr. 1/200, and you have on hand gr. 1/300 tablets. To obtain the dosage of gr. 1/200 in 15 minims of finished solution, you must dissolve _____ tablet (s) in _____ minims of diluent.

14

14

5 minims

When you have dissolved 2 of the gr. 1/300 tablets in 20 minims of diluent, and you are supposed to give 15 minims, you must discard _____ minims before giving the injection.

UNIT III
STOCK SOLUTIONS

1

50 mg. : 1 ml

1

In some instances, the drug on hand is already in solution and the amount of drug per milliliter is written on the label of the vial. A label reading "50 mg. per ml." tells you that the ratio of milligrams to milliliters is_____ : _____.

2

35 mg.: X ml.

2

Since the drug is already in solution, the nurse does not need to determine the amount of diluent to use. The unknown factor is the amount of solution to be given so that the correct dosage is obtained. The label on the vial gives us our first ratio.

Our second ratio shows the amount of drug ordered by the physician compared to the amount to be given in milliliters. If the physician orders 35 mg., our second ratio would be_____ mg.:_____ ml.

3

0.7 ml.

3

If a physician orders 35 mg. of Demerol and the label on the multiple-dose vial reads 50 mg. per ml., the proportion is written:

50 mg. : 1 ml. = 35 mg. : X ml.

The amount of solution to be given is _____.

4

10.5 minims

4

Some syringes are calibrated in minims rather than tenths of a milliliter. To give the patient 0.7 ml. (or 0.7 of 15 minims), the nurse should pull the plunger of the syringe back to the line marked_____minims.

Arithmetically, the correct answer to the question in Frame 4 is 10.5 minims, but a minim is such a small amount that the number 10.5 should be rounded off to 11.

5

1.5 cc.

5

You are instructed to give 37.5 mg. of Leritine. The label on the 2-cc. ampule reads 50 mg. The patient should be given _____cc. of the drug.

If you had no trouble finding the correct answer to the problem in Frame 5, go on to Frame 7. If you did not get the right answer, go on to Frame 6.

6

1.5 cc.

6

You probably missed the problem because you failed to notice that the ratio of drug to solution was 50 mg.:2cc., rather than 50 mg.:1 cc.

Be very careful when you are reading labels on medication!

Your proportion should be:

50 mg. : 2 cc. = 37.5 mg. : X cc.

When you solve for X, you find that the patient should receive_____cc.

7

7

20 minims

Let's say that you have a 2-cc, ampule of caffeine sodium benzoate, and that the ampule contains gr. viiss. If physician orders gr. v, you should give the patient _____ minims.

Surely you didn't miss this one! If you did, go back and look at the question again. We asked for the number of minims to be given.

8

8

10 minims

Suppose that a physician orders gr. 1/6 of morphine sulfate. The drug is available in a multiple-dose vial labeled 15 mg. per cc. How many minims should the patient receive? _____

If you did not have the correct answer to the problem in Frame 8, go on to Frame 9. If you were right, go on to Frame 11.

9

9

10 mg.

You seem to be forgetting that you must convert when a drug is ordered in one system and the supply on hand is in another system. We convert the dosage ordered by the physician into the units of the dosage on hand.

To determine the equivalent in milligrams for 1/6 grain, you write the proportion:

60 mg. : 1 gr. = X mg. : 1/6 gr.

When you solve for X, you find that 1/6 grain = _____ mg.

10

10 minims

10

The physician ordered 10 mg. and the dosage on hand is 15 mg. per cc. To determine the number of minims to be given the patient, you must change the cubic centimeters to minims. If 1 cc. = 15 minims, your proportion is:

15 mg. : 15 minims = 10 mg. : X minims

When you solve for X, you find that the patient should receive_____minims.

11

15 minims

11

Suppose that a physician orders atropine 0.4 mg. The drug is available in a multiple-dose vial labeled gr. 1/150 per cc. You should give the patient_____minims of atropine.

12

3 minims

12

Let's say that you have been instructed to give a patient 0.25 mg. of Serpasil. The drug is dispensed in 2-cc. ampules containing 2.5 mg. The patient should receive _____minims of the drug.

UNIT IV

DRUGS MEASURED IN UNITS

1

cannot

1

Most drugs are standardized. This means that their active ingredients can be separated and chemically analyzed. Since the active chemical ingredients of these drugs are known, they can be measured according to the standard systems of measurement.

There are some drugs, however, that cannot be analyzed chemically. Since we cannot separate the active ingredients of these drugs, they   ·   can / cannot   ·
be measured according to the usual systems of measurement.

2

units

2

Drugs that cannot be analyzed by chemical means are standardized according to their effect on laboratory animals. These drugs are labeled in *units*. The word *"unit"* in this sense means the amount needed to bring about the desired effect in a laboratory animal. The strength of hormones, vitamins, and some other drugs must be determined by their effects on laboratory animals. These medications are labeled in_____.

3

3

standards

All drugs must meet certain standards. When we see the words "U.S.P. Units" on a label, this means that the drug meets the _____ set by the United States Pharmacopeia.

4

4

diluent

Drugs that are labeled in units may be in solid or liquid form. If a drug comes in solid form, the nurse must read the directions on the accompanying circular provided by the manufacturer to determine the amount of diluent to add to obtain correct dosage.

When a solid drug is measured in units, the nurse must read the accompanying directions to find the amount of · diluent / units. · needed.

5

5

solution

Sometimes drugs that are labeled in units are already in solution when dispensed from the pharmacy. Since a diluent does not need to be added, the nurse sets up a proportion for the purpose of determining the amount of solution to be given.

When a drug is already in solution, we use ratio and proportion to determine the amount of _____ to be given so that the desired dosage is obtained.

6

units : ml.

6

The procedure for setting up the proportion for drugs already in solution is the same whether the drug is measured in grams or labeled in units. If the drug is labeled in grams, the ratio will be Gm: ml. If the drug is labeled in units, the first ratio will be:

_____ : _____

7

40 units : 1 ml.
= 50 units : X ml.

7

The first ratio represents the dosage on hand and is expressed units : ml. The second ratio represents dosage ordered in units: amount of solution to be given.

Let's suppose that you have on hand a vial containing 40 units per ml., and a physician orders 50 units. The proportion would be:

_____ : _____ = _____ : _____

8

1.25 ml.

8

Your proportion is 40 units : 1 ml. = 50 units: X ml. When you solve for X, you find that the patient should receive _____ of the soultion.

9

12 minims

9

If a physician orders 8000 units of heparin and the dosage on hand is 10,000 units per cc., the patient should receive_____ minims.

10

9 minims

10

Let's say a physician orders Chymar 3000 units. The drug is dispensed in vials of 5000 units per ml. The patient should receive _____ minims.

11

1.3 cc.

11

If you were asked to give a patient 400,000 units of penicillin, and the drug was available only in a multiple-dose vial containing 300,000 units per cc., you would give the patient _____ cc. of the drug.

12

1.5 ml.

12

A physician orders 60 units of ACTH to be given I.M., and the dosage on hand is 40 units per ml. The amount that you would give the patient is _____ ml.

UNIT V

CALCULATING INSULIN DOSAGE

1

units

1

Insulin is a hormone secreted by the Islands of Langerhans—which are small, scattered masses of cells on the surface of the pancreas. Since the active ingredients of this hormone have not been analyzed completely, insulin dosage must be prescribed in units.

Commercial preparations of insulin are standardized according to their effect on laboratory animals, and therefore are labeled in _____.

2

label

2

Insulin comes in various strengths and types. Each vial of insulin is plainly labeled as to its strength and type. Before attempting to calculate any dosage of insulin, the nurse must carefully read the_____on the vial she is using.

3

80 units

3

The most commonly used strengths of insulin are U.40 and U.80. The designation U.40 means that there are 40 units of insulin per cubic centimeter in the vial. Thus, U.80 on a label means that there are_____ units of insulin per cc.

4

U.80

5

U.40

4

The reason for having insulin in different strengths is to allow for the administration of not more than 1 cc. per dose. If, for example, a patient is to receive 50 units of insulin, it would be best to use •
U.40/U.80 • insulin for this injection.

5

The easiest and most accurate method of measuring insulin is by using an insulin syringe. The drawing shows how most insulin syringes are calibrated to ensure accurate dosage.

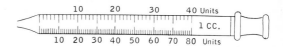

One side of the scale on the syringe is calibrated for the administration of U.40 insulin. The other side is calibrated for U.80 insulin. If a nurse is to give 30 units of insulin, and the vial is labeled U.40 insulin, she would read the side of the scale calibrated for_____insulin.

6

should not

6

Insulin is also available in strengths of U.20 and U.100. Although these strengths are not used so often as U.40 and U.80 insulin, the nurse must be aware that they are available. It is obvious that if the insulin is labeled U.20 or U.100, the best way to measure a dose of this strength would be by using a syringe calibrated for the administration of U.20 or U.100 insulin.

If a nurse is giving insulin from a vial labeled U.100, she · should/should not · use an insulin syringe calibrated for U.40 and U.80 insulin.

7

one

7

There are times when an insulin syringe is not available or when the one available is not calibrated according to the strength of the insulin on hand. If the dosage is simply one ml. (as for example when giving 40 units of U.40 insulin) the nurse may use any type of syringe calibrated in ml. or cc. If the physician orders 80 units of insulin and the nurse is using U.80 insulin, she can use any type of syringe and give the patient _____ ml. of the drug.

8

20 units:1 ml.

8

Sometimes the nurse finds that she must give less than 1 ml. of insulin. She then uses ratio and proportion to determine the fractional dose. Her first ratio will be the strength of the insulin. The ratio of U.20 insulin per ml. is:

_____units:_____ml.

9

20 units:1 ml.=
15 units:X ml.

9

The first ratio indicates the units of insulin per milliliter in the vial on hand. The second ratio shows the relation between the dosage ordered by the physician and the unknown number of milliliters (X) to be given.

If the physician orders 15 units of insulin and the drug on hand is U.20 insulin, the proportion is written:

_____:_____ = _____:_____

10

0.75 ml.

10

Solving for X, she finds that the patient should receive_____ml. of U.20 insulin in order to give 15 units.

11

11

tuberculin

In the preceding problem you found that 0.75 ml. of U.20 insulin must be given. Let us say an insulin syringe calibrated for U.20 insulin is not available. A tuberculin syringe calibrated in tenths and hundredths of a ml. is available. Since the dosage is 0.75 ml., it would be possible to use a _____ syringe for measuring the correct dose.

12

12

minims

When you set up your proportion in the preceding problem, X represented the number of ml. to be given. Since you had a tuberculin syringe calibrated in hundredths of a ml., no further calculation was necessary. If, however, you had decided to use a syringe calibrated in minims, you would need to determine the number of_____ to give the patient.

13

13

3.75 minims

0.25 ml.

Let's say that a physician orders 5 units of insulin. The drug on hand is U.20 insulin. The nurse would give the patient_____ minims or _____ ml.

Remember that 3.75 minims is a very small amount, and should be rounded off to 4 minims.

14

12.75 minims
(13 minims)
or 8.5 ml.

15

11 minims
0.75 ml.

16

7 minims
0.4 ml.

17

14 minims
0.9 ml.

14

You are instructed to give a patient 85 units of insulin, and you have on hand U.100 insulin. You would give the patient _____ minims, or_____ml.

15

Suppose that a physician orders 30 units of insulin, and that the drug is dispensed in a vial of U.40 insulin. If you found that no insulin syringe was available, you would give the patient_____minims, or_____ ml.

16

If a physician orders 35 units of insulin, and the drug is available in U.80 strength, the patient should be given_____minims or _____ml.

17

Let's say that a physician orders 75 units of insulin, and the drug is available only in U.80 strength. If she has no insulin syringe, the nurse should convert this dosage to _____minims or_____ml.

POST-TEST ON PREPARING SOLUTIONS FOR PARENTERAL ADMINISTRATION

A. Situations

1. Directions accompanying an injectable powdered drug read as follows: *Add 1.7 ml. of diluent (each ml. will contain 500 mg.).* In order to give 0.5 Gm. of the drug the nurse would give_____ml. of the solution.

2. A nurse must give 0.25 Gm. of an antibiotic. Directions accompanying the drug read: *Add 8.6 ml. of diluent (each ml. contains 500 mg.).* After adding the diluent the nurse would give the patient_____ml. of the solution.

3. The dosage on hand is a hypodermic tablet of gr. 1/100. The dosage desired is gr. 1/150. How much diluent would be used to obtain the correct amount of drug in 1 ml.?
_____

4. The dosage desired is gr. 1/4. The hypodermic tablets on hand contain gr. 1/6 each. How many tablets would be used?_____. How much dilueunt would be used to obtain the correct dosage in one ml.?_____.

5. The physician orders 30 mg. of Demerol. The drug on hand is a vial labeled "50 mg. per cc." How many minims would be given to obtain the correct dosage?_____

6. The dosage on hand is 50 mg. per 2 cc. The physician orbers 37.5 mg. How many cc. of stock solution would you give the patient?_____

7. The physician orders 0.8 mg. of Levo-Dromoran. The drug on hand is a vial ladeled 2 mg. per cc. How many minims

of solution would be given? _____ .

8. A physician orders gr. 1/300 of a certain drug. The dosage on hand is a hypodermic tablet of gr. 1/200 each. How much diluent would be used to dissolve the tablet so that the correct dosage is obtained in one ml.? _____

9. The dosage ordered is 35 units of insulin. Using a 2 cc. or tuberculin syringe and a vial of U.40 insulin, you would give the patient _____ minims or _____ ml.

10. A physician orders 60 units of insulin and the dosage on hand is U.80 insulin. If the insulin is measured in a 2 cc. or tuberculin syringe, you would give the patient _____ minims or _____ ml.

PART SEVEN

PREPARING LARGE AMOUNTS OF SOLUTIONS

UNIT I

PURE DRUGS

1

nurse

1

In most large hopsitals, the solutions used for irrigations and other treatments are prepared in the pharmacy or in the central supply department, and the pharmacist determines the amount of drug to use to obtain a solution of correct strength. The nurse, however, must also know how to make these solutions.

In many smaller hospitals there is no pharmacist on the staff, and the _____ may be the person responsible for preparing the solutions needed for various treatments.

2

liquid

2

Solutions may be prepared from pure drugs or from strong stock solutions. In this unit, we will be concerned only with pure drugs. When we speak of pure drugs, we mean unadulterated substances in solid or liquid form. Making a solution from a pure drug involves dissolving a solid substance, or diluting a _____ substance.

3

3

proportion

There are several different ways to determine the amount of pure drug to use in preparing a solution of a certain strength. Since you are familiar with ratio and proportion, we will use this method.

To prepare a solution from a pure drug, the nurse may determine the amount of pure drug needed by finding the value of an unknown in a _____.

4

4

pure drug

In a proportion, the letter X represents the unknown factor. When you are using a proportion to find the amount of pure drug needed to prepare a given amount of solution, the X represents the amount of _____ required.

5

5

pure drug
finished solution

When you prepare a solution, you must first decide how much of the finished solution you will need. The first ratio of the proportion will show the amount of pure drug contained in this amount of finished solution.

The first ratio of the proportion will be: amount of _____ _____ : known   amount   of _____

_____.

6

5:100

6

In addition to knowing the amount of fin-ished solution you will need, you must also know the strength desired for this solution. This strength is the second ratio of the proportion.

Let's say that you will need a 5% solution. The term "5%" means that there will be 5 parts of a substance in every 100 parts of the solution. Expressed as a ratio, 5% is the same as:

_____ : _____

7

X : 1000 =
5:100

7

Now we can see that a proportion can be set up for a situation in which we need to prepare 1000 ml. of a 5% solution. We will use the proportion to determine the amount of pure drug needed. The proportion will express, X parts of pure drug: _____ parts of finished solution = _____ parts: _____ parts.

8

grams

8

We know that we must use units of measure to express the parts or amounts needed for the solution and the pure drug. The gram and the milliliter are the acceptable equivalents for solids and liquids, respectively.

The finished solution will be measured in milliliters. The pure drug in liquid form will be measured in milliliters. The pure drug in solid form will be measured in _____ .

9

5 Gm. : 100 ml.

Now you may ask how we can compare grams to milliliters in one ratio and then compare a percentage to 100 in the other ratio. Actually, the term "5% solution" means that there are to be 5 Gm. or 5 ml. of the pure drug in every 100 ml. of diluent. A 5% solution made from a solid pure drug can be written as the ratio:

_____ Gm.: _____ ml.

10

X Gm. : 2000 ml =
2 Gm. : 100 ml.

Now let's see how we set up a proportion for another situation. Suppose that you must prepare 2000 ml. of a 2% solution using boric acid crystals.

Because the pure drug is a solid, the proportion will compare grams to milliliters and will be written:

_____ : _____ = _____ : _____

11

40 Gm.

You solve for X to find how much pure drug should be used in 2000 ml. so that there will be 2 Gm. in every 100 ml. Your proportion is X Gm. : 2000 ml. = 2 Gm. : 100 ml.

The amount of pure drug needed for 2000 ml. is _____ Gm.

12

X Gm. :1000 ml. =
2.5 Gm. :100 ml.

12

Suppose that a physician orders compresses using a 2 1/2% solution of maganesium sulfate. You will need to prepare 1 quart of this solution. Your proportion for this would be:

_____ : _____ = _____ : _____

    If you set up the correct proportion for the problem in Frame 12, go on to Frame 15. If you did not get the right proportion, go on to Frame 13.

13

metric
metric

13

Solutions may be ordered according to the apothecaries' system, but the _____ system is the one most often used for weighing and measuring drugs because of its accuracy. When a solution is ordered in the apothecaries' system, the amount of finished solution should be converted to the _____ system.

14

1000 ml.

14

Since the physician has ordered 1 quart of a 2 1/2% solution, we must convert 1 quart to _____ before setting up the proportion.

15

5 Gm.

15

In another situation, a physician orders warm saline gargles using a 1% solution. The amount of sodium chloride needed to prepare 1 pint of solution would be

_____.

16

5 Gm.

16

Another time, you find that you must prepare 2000 ml. of a 1/4% solution. The pure drug is in solid form.

After setting up your proportion and solving for X, you find that you will need _____ of pure drug.

17

X ml. : 4000 ml.
= 2 ml. : 100 ml.

17

Cresol solution is frequently used as a disinfectant. The solution is prepared from a pure liquid drug. If you needed to prepare 1 gallon of a 2% solution of cresol, your proportion would be:

_____ : _____ = _____ : _____

18

80 ml.

18

Solving for X, you find that to prepare 1 gallon of a 2% cresol solution you will need _____ ml. of the pure drug.

19

X Gm. : 2000 ml. =
1 Gm. : 1000 ml.

19

Sometimes the strength of a solution is ordered as a ratio, such as 1:1000. In this case, your second ratio is already set up for you. Let's say you needed 2000 ml. of a 1:1000 solution. Your proportion is written:
_____ Gm.: _____ ml. = _____ Gm.: _____ ml.

20

2 Gm.

20

After solving for X, you find that to prepare 2000 ml. of a 1:1000 solution, you will need _____ Gm. of pure drug.

21

40 ml.

21

Let's suppose that the nurse must prepare 1 gallon of a 1:100 solution. The pure drug is available in liquid form. She would use _____ of pure drug.

22

3960 ml.

22

When preparing solutions, the correct procedure is to put the pure drug in a graduated container and add to it enough of the diluent to produce the desired amount of finished solution.

In a previous situation, you used 40 ml. of pure drug to make a solution. The amount of diluent needed to make this a 4000-ml. finished solution would be_____ ml.

23

23

8 Gm.

To prepare 80 ml. of a 10% solution, a nurse would need to use_____ of pure drug in solid form.

24

24

24 tablets

Let's say that you must make 0.4 liters of a 3% solution. You have on hand a pure drug in the form of 0.5 Gm. tablets. To prepare the solution, you would use _____ tablet(s).

If you answered the question in Frame 24 without difficulty, go on to Frame 27. If you did not completely understand how we got the answer, go on to Frame 25 for an explanation.

25

25

400 ml.

You will recall that a 3% solution means that there are 3 Gm. or 3 ml. of solute for every 100 ml. of solution. Since the second ratio of the proportion compares grams to milli- liters, the first ratio must also compare grams to milliliters.

The correct ratio for X grams to 0.4 liters would be:

X Gm.:_____ml.

26

24 tablets

26

Your proportion is now X Gm. : 400 ml. = 3 Gm. : 100 ml. When you solve for X, you find that you will need 12 Gm. of the pure drug. To obtain 12 Gm. from the 0.5 Gm. tablets, you would need to use_____ tablet(s).

27

2 Gm.

27

Suppose that you wish to prepare 2000 ml. of a 1 : 1000 solution from 5 gr. tablets. Using the proportion X Gm. : 2000 ml. = 1 Gm. : 1000 ml., you find that you will need _____Gm. of pure drug.

28

30 grains
6 tablets

28

In this problem, the pure drug was available in 5 gr. tablets. If you need 2 Gm., this would be the same as_____grain(s) or_____ tablet(s).

29

1 tablet

29

To prepare 1 liter of a 1:2000 solution, using gr. viiss. tablets, the nurse would have to use _____tablet(s).

30

100 ml.

3900 ml.

30

Suppose that the pure drug on hand is a liquid, and that you need to prepare 4 liters of a 2 1/2% solution.

You would use_____ml. of pure drug and_____ml. of diluent.

31

31

36 Gm.

The strength of physiological saline (normal saline) is 0.9%. To prepare 1 gallon of normal saline using sodium chloride crystals, a nurse would need_____Gm. of the pure drug.

32

32

1%

A 5% solution means that there are 5 parts of one substance in every 100 parts of the solution. If you used 10 Gm. of pure drug in 1000 ml. of solution, you would have 10 parts of pure drug in every 1000 parts of solution. This is a ratio of 10:1000, or 1:100. Expressed as a percentage, this would be _____%.

33

33

8%

Let's say that you have used 80 ml. of pure drug in 1000 ml. of solution. The ratio would be 80 : 1000. The percentage of your finished solution would be_____%.

UNIT II
STOCK SOLUTIONS

1

stock

1

The preceding problems were concerned with the preparation of solutions from a pure drug. Sometimes, however, a nurse must prepare solutions from a strong stock solution.

Hospitals keep on hand concentrated solutions from which various strengths of weaker solutions can be made. These strong solutions are called _____ solutions because they are always kept on hand.

2

less

2

We do not use the same proportion for stock solutions as for pure drugs. When we use a strong stock solution to make a weaker solution, we are dealing with two different strengths. The strength of the finished solution will be · less / greater · than the strength of the stock solution.

3

lesser
greater

3

Our proportion for stock solutions compares amounts of the solutions as well as their strengths. The first ratio compares the lesser amount to the greater amount. The second ratio must follow the same order and compare the _____ strength to the _____ strength.

4

X ml. : 1000 ml
= 2% : 4%

4

Now we have our proportion for preparing a weaker solution from a strong stock solution. The lesser amount of stock solution is to the greater amount of stock solution as the lesser strength is to the greater strength.

   If you need to prepare 1000 ml. of a 2% solution from a 4% stock solution, your proportion would be:

X ml.:_____ml. = _____%
        :_____ %

5

stock solution

5

Your proportion is set up to determine the amount of stock solution to use. It is written X ml.:1000 ml.=2% : 4%. You solve for X, and find that 500 ml. is the amount of _____ _____ to be used.

6

500 ml.

6

Your problem was to prepare 1000 ml. of finished solution. If you used 500 ml. of stock solution, the amount of diluent to be added would be_____.

7

X ml. : 500 ml
= 2% : 10%

7

Suppose that you needed to prepare 1 pint of a 2% solution from a 10% stock solution. Your proportion for this would be:

_____ : _____ = _____ : _____

8

100 ml.
400 ml.

8

Your proportion is X ml. : 500 ml. $= 2\%$: 10%. When you solve for X, you find that the amount of stock solution needed is _____ and the amount of diluent to be added is _____.

9

75 cc.
675 cc

9

Let's say that a nurse needs 750 cc. of a 5% solution. The stock solution on hand is a 50% solution. To make 750 cc. of finished solution, she would pour _____ of stock solution into a graduated pitcher and add _____ of diluent.

10

1 part
1000 parts

10

The strength of a stock solution may be expressed by a percentage or by a ratio. Zephiran Chloride, for example, is available in strengths of 1:1000, 1:3000, and so forth.

A 1:1000 solution would have _____ part(s) of Zephiran Chloride in every _____ parts of finished solution.

11

1/3000

11

When the strength of a stock solution is expressed in a ratio, it is necessary to change the ratio to a fraction before setting up the proportion. The ratio of 1:3000 can be written as the common fraction _____.

12

1/3000:1/1000

12

You know that the proportion for preparing a weaker solution from a stronger solution is lesser amount : greater amount = lesser strength : greater strength. If you were to prepare a 1:3000 solution from a 1:1000 solution, the second ratio would be set up as_____ :_____.

If you missed the proportion in Frame 12, you probably forgot that the larger the denominator of a fraction, the less the value of the fraction. Remember that 1/8 of a pie is a smaller slice than 1/4 of a pie.

13

X cc. : 500 cc.
   = 1/3000
   : 1/1000

13

Now let's see how we would set up the entire proportion in a nursing situation. You must prepare 500 cc. of a 1:3000 solution, and the stock solution on hand is 1:1000. Your proportion would be:

_____cc.:_____cc. = _____:_____

14

167 cc.
333 cc.

14

When you calculate X, you find that you must use_____of stock solution and add_____of diluent to make 500 cc. of finished solution.

15

15

Let's say that a nurse needs to prepare 1/2 gallon of a 1 : 20 solution. The stock solution on hand is 1 : 5 strength.

stock solution
diluent

When you solve for X, you find that the amount of_____ _____
used would be 500 cc. and the amount of _____ added would be 1500 cc.

16

400 ml.
600 ml.

16

A nurse needs to prepare 1 liter of a 1:500 solution. The stock solution is labeled 1:200. She would have to mix _____ of stock solution with _____ of diluent.

17

5:100

17

Up to this point we have worked problems in which the strength of the solution desired and the strength of the solution on hand were both expressed in the same manner, either as a percentage or as a ratio.

There are times, however, when the two strengths are expressed in different terms— one as a percentage and the other as a ratio. In this case we cannot set up a proportion until both strengths are expressed in like terms. Therefore, we must either change the percentage to a ratio or change the ratio to a percentage.

It does not matter which change we make, so long as both strengths are finally expressed in like terms. You already know that it is simple to change a percentage to a ratio: 5% means 5 parts per 100, and can be expressed as the ratio_____:_____.

18

18

1/10%

To change a ratio to a percentage, you must first realize that a ratio can be written as a fraction. Once the ratio has been changed to a fraction, it can be changed to percentage by multiplying by 100. Thus the ratio 1:1000 becomes the fraction 1/1000, and 1/1000 × 100 = _____%.

19

19

(a) 8.33%
(b) 25%
(c) 2%
(d) 40%
(e) 4%

A nurse should be quite proficient in changing ratios to percentages. See if you can work the following problems without difficulty:

    (a) 1:12 = _____ %
    (b) 8:32 = _____ %
    (c) 1:50 = _____ %
    (d) 2:5 = _____ %
    (e) 3:75 = _____ %

20

20

X ml : 3000 ml.
  = 1 / 4000:
      2 / 100

Now let's say that you need to prepare 3 liters of a 1:4000 solution from a 2% stock solution. If you changed 2% to a fraction, your proportion would be:
    X ml.: _____ = _____ : _____

21

21

X ml. : 3000 ml.
  =1 / 40%
    : 2%

If you changed the ratio of 1 : 4000 to a percentage, your proportion would be:

    X ml.: _____ = _____ : _____

22

37.5 ml.

22

No matter whether you change the percentage to a ratio or the ratio to a percentage, when you solve for X you will find that you need_____ml. of the stock solution.

23

400 ml.

23

Suppose that you need 1/2 gallon of a 1:50 solution, and the stock solution on hand is 10%. After setting up your proportion and solving for X, you find that you will need to use_____of stock solution.

24

250 ml.
750 ml.

24

If you need to prepare 1000 ml. of a 1% solution, and the stock solution on hand is 1:25 strength, you would use _____ of stock solution and _____ of diluent.

25

1000 ml.

25

A physician orders compresses using a 1:20 solution. You will need to prepare 1 gallon of the solution. The stock solution on hand is 20% strength. The amount of stock solution you would use is _____.

26

3000 ml.

26

Then, to prepare 1 gallon of the finished solution, you would add_____ of diluent to the 1000 ml. of stock solution.

POST-TEST ONE PREPARING LARGE AMOUNT OF SOLUTIONS

A. Situations:

1. To prepare 1 gallon of a 4 % solution from cresol, which is a pure drug in liquid form, you would use _____ of pure drug and _____ of diluent.

2. To prepare 1000 ml. of a 4 % solution from a pure drug in solid form, you would need _____ of pure drug.

3. To prepare 2 gallons of a 1:1000 solution from a pure drug in liquid form, you would need _____ of pure drug.

4. To prepare 1 pint of a 0.9% solution from a 10 % stock solution, you would use _____ of stock solution in _____ of diluent.

5. To prepare 2 liters of a 1:2000 solution from a 2% stock solution, you would need _____ of stock solution and _____ of diluent.

ANSWERS TO THE POST-TEST QUESTIONS

PART ONE
INTRODUCTION TO SYSTEMS OF MEASUREMENT

Completion

1. system
2. apothecaries', metric
3. household
4. metric
5. apothecaries.'

PART TWO
THE APOTHECARIES' SYSTEM

A.   Table of equivalents

1. 60 minims
2. 8 drams
3. 16 ounces
4. 2 pints
5. 32 ounces
6. 4 quarts

B. Abbreviations

1. gal.
2. qt.
3. pt.
4. oz.
5. dr.
6. gr.

C. Symbols

1. ℥
2. ℨ
3. ℳ

D. Reading dosages

1. Two and one-half ounces
2. Four ounces
3. Two drams
4. One-half ounce
5. Eight drams
6. Thirteen minims
7. Seven minims
8. Seven and one-half grains
9. Twenty grains
10. Fifteen grains

E. Charting dosages

1. Mineral oil ℥ iii
2. Cascara ℨ iss.
3. Tincture of belladonna ℳxv
4. Elixir of Donnatal ℨ ss.
5. Aspirin gr. v

F. Situations

1. 2 quarts   1/2 gallon
2. No.
3. No.
4. minim glass or 2 cc. syringe
5. 4 5/12 grains
6. 1/64 grain
7. 3 3/4 grains

8. 1/8 grain
9. 1/75 grain
10. 2 tablets

THREE
THE HOUSEHOLD SYSTEM

Situations

1. 1 ounce
2. 1 tablespoonful
3. 1 tablespoonful
4. 2 bottles

PART FOUR
THE METRIC SYSTEM

A. Table of equivalents

1. 1000 ml.
2. 1 cc.
3. 1000 mg.

B. Abbreviations

1. L.
2. Gm.
3. ml.
4. mg.
5. cc.

C. Reading metric abbreviations

1. Thirty-five hundredths milligram
2. Two-tenths milligram

3. One and seventy-five hundredths milligrams
4. Five-tenths gram
5. Six-tenths milliliter
6. Fifty-five hundredths liter
7. Two and five-tenths milliliters
8. Four-hundredths milligram
9. Four and eight-tenths liters
10. Seven and five-tenths grams

D. Charting dosages

1. 1.5 Gm.
2. 0.3 mg.
3. 0.07 ml.
4. 0.75 L.
5. 2.5 mg.

E. Situations

1. 2 bottles
2. 3 tablets
3. 6 tablets
4. 1 tablet
5. 10 cc.
    0.4 Gm.
6. 5 tablets
7. 2 tablets
8. 8 cc.
    5 days
9. 2 capsules
10. 200 mg.
    1 tablet

PART FIVE
EXCHANGING UNITS OF WEIGHT AND MEASURE BETWEEN THE APOTHECARIES' AND THE METRIC SYSTEMS

A. Table of equivalents

1. 2 liters
2. 4 liters
3. 2000 ml.
4. 2 pints
5. 30 ml.
6. 2 drams
7. 30 minims
8. 10 minims
9. 1 1/3 ml.
10. 2 ml.
11. 0.02 Gm.
12. 0.5 Gm.
13. 3 3/4 grains
14. 30 grains
15. 3 grains

B. Situations

1. 2 L.
2. 4 ml.
   gr. ii ss
3. gr. iii.
4. 2 tablets
5. 6 tablets
6. 1 tablet
7. 2 tablets
8. 3 tablets
9. 2 tablets
10. 1/2 tablet

PART SIX
PREPARING SOLUTIONS FOR PARENTERAL ADMINISTRATION

A. Situations

1. 1 ml.
2. 0.5 ml.
3. 1.5 ml.
4. 2 tablets
   1.3 ml.
5. 9 minims
6. 1.5 ml.
7. 6 minims
8. 1.5 ml.
9. 13 minims or 0.9 ml.
10. 11 minims or 0.8 ml.

PART SEVEN
PREPARING LARGE AMOUNTS OF SOLUTIONS

A. Situations

1. 160 ml. of pure drug; 3840 ml. of diluent
2. 40 Gm. of pure drug
3. 8 ml. of pure drug
4. 45 ml. of stock solution; 455 ml. of diluent
5. 50 ml. of stock solution; 1950 ml. of diluent

EXAMINATION

1. A patient with severe contact dermatitis is to receive cold compresses of Burow's solution (aluminum acetate) in a 1:20 dilution 4 times per day. If ℥ xvi of solution are needed for each application,_____ qt(s) will be necessary each day. This is the same as _____ gal. (s).

2. Mrs. Zolot is receiving 4 ml. of camphorated tincture of opium (paregoric). If each dose is diluted with water to make ℥ i, the nurse will add ℥ _____ of water to the medication.

3. The medication card reads "Tincture of belladonna ♏x." If the patient receives this amount 3 times a day, he receives a total of ℥ _____.

4. The doctor has ordered gr. 1/300. If the drug is available in tablets of gr. 1/150 and gr. 1/600, you would give the patient · two gr. 1/150 tablets / two gr. 1/600 tablets.

5. Phenprocoumor (Liquamar) is an anticoagulant that is given in varying dosages, adjusted for each individual patient. Let us say that Mr. Good received 21 mg. the first day, 7.5 mg. the second day, 3 mg. the third day, and 0.25 mg. the fourth day. What is the total amount of Liquamar received by Mr. Good in four days? _____.

6. The initial dose of methylchlothiazide may be as much as 0.01 Gm. daily. If you have this drug avail-

able in tablets labeled 5 mg., how many tablets should be given for an initial dose of 0.01 Gm.? _____ .

7. A 3 year old girl is to receive Furoxone 0.033 Gm. 4 times daily. The drug is available in an oral suspension of 16.6 mg./5 ml. How many ml. would the child receive for each dose? _____ .

8. A patient with severe myasthenia gravis is to receive Mestinon syrup 0.36 Gm. The dosage on hand is 60 mg./5 ml. How many ml. should he receive? _____ How many ounces is this? _____ .

9. Dimetane is available in elixir labeled 2 mg./5 ml. How much Dimetane is contained in each ml.? _____ .

10. A child who is a clinic patient is to receive 2 teaspoonfuls of Vi-daylin each day. In order to provide a 30-day supply, the patient's mother should receive a · 3 ounce / 8 ounce / pint · bottle to take home.

11. A patient with angina pectoris is receiving nitroglycerin gr. 1/600 as needed for pain. The label on the bottle is 0.1 mg. You should give the patient _____ tablet(s) to provide the dosage of gr. 1/600.

12. The doctor has ordered quinidine sulfate gr. vi. and it is dispensed in tablets of 0.2 Gm. each. You should give _____ tablet(s).

13. A patient is to receive diethylstilbestrol gr. 1/120 and the drug is available is 0.25 mg. tablets. How many tablets should the patient receive? _____ .

14. The doctor has ordered Sodium Nembutal gr. ss intramuscularly. The drug is available in an ampule containing 100 mg./2 ml. You should give the patient _____ minims.

15. A pediatric patient is to receive 0.06 Gm. of Kantrex Pediatric Injection. It is dispensed in vials of 75 mg./2 ml. The patient should receive _____ ml.

16. You have on hand a 4.0 Gm. vial of Staphcillin, and the

physician has ordered 1.0 Gm. Directions accompanying the vial read as follows: *Add 5.7 ml. diluent (each 1 ml. contains 500 mg. Staphcillin)*. After adding the diluent you should administer _____ml. to the patient.

17. A physician orders gr. 1/8 and the dosage on hand is a gr. 1/6 hypodermic tablet. To give the patient 15 minims containing gr. 1/8, the nurse should dissolve the gr. 1/6 tablet in_____minims of diluent and discard_____minims of solution before giving the injection.

18. A child on the pediatric ward is to receive 3 mg. of Vasoxyl. You have on hand an ampule labeled 10 mg./cc. How many ml. should the child receive? _____. If a tuberculin syringe is not available, how many minims should be given?_____.

19. A pediatric patient is to receive gr. 1/250 of scopolamine as a preoperative medication. The drug on hand is a vial labeled gr. 1/200 per ml. The patient should receive_____minims.

20. The physician has ordered 6000 units of heparin. The drug is dispensed in an ampule labeled 10,000 units per cc. The patient should receive_____cc. or_____minims.

21. Suppose that you were teaching a diabetic patient about insulin. In explaining the difference between U.40 and U.80 insulin, you could say that U.40 was · half as strong / twice as strong · as U.80 insulin.

22. A patient is to receive 60 units of insulin. The drug on hand is U.80 insulin. The nurse should administer _____ml. or_____minims.

23. In order to prepare one pint of normal saline (0.9%) solution for a throat irrigation, the nurse would need _____Gm. of pure drug (sodium chloride crystals).

24. To prepare 3 quarts of a 1:1000 solution from pure drug in liquid form, you would need_____ml. of pure drug and_____ml. of diluent.

25. You must prepare 2 liters of a 1:2000 solution from a 4% stock solution. You will use_____ml. of the stock solution and add_____ml. of diluent.

ANSWERS TO THE EXAMINATION QUESTIONS

1. 2 quarts
    1/2 gallon
2. ℥ vii
3. ℥ ss
4. two gr. 1/600 tablets
5. 31.75 mg.
6. 2 tablets
7. 10 ml.
8. 30 ml.
    1 ounce
9. 0.4 mg.
10. 8 ounces
11. 1 tablet
12. 2 tablets
13. 2 tablets
14. 9 minims
15. 1.6 ml.
16. 2 ml.
17. 20 minims of diluent; discard 5 minims
18. 0.3 ml.
    4.5 minims
19. 12 minims
20. 0.6 cc.
    9 minims
21. half as strong

22. 0.8 ml.
    11 minims
23. 4.5 Gm.
24. 3 ml. of pure drug
    2997 ml. of diluent
25. 25 ml. of stock solution
    1975 ml. of diluent